T0316475

# THE ULTIMATE GUIDE TO BONDAGE

# THE ULTIMATE GUIDE TO BONDAGE

## CREATING INTIMACY THROUGH THE ART OF RESTRAINT

By Mistress Couple

CLEiS PRESS

Published in the United States by Cleis Press, an imprint of Start Midnight, LLC, 101 Hudson Street, Thirty-Seventh Floor, Suite 3705, Jersey City, NJ 07302.

Printed in the United States.
Cover design: Allyson Fields
Cover photograph: Kiki Vassilakis
Illustrations: Emily Dorr
Text design: Frank Wiedemann
First Edition.
10 9 8 7 6 5 4 3 2 1

Trade paper ISBN: 978-1-62778- 274-6
E-book ISBN: 978-1-62778-275-3

Library of Congress Cataloging-in-Publication Data is available on file.

# CONTENTS


| | | |
|---|---|---|
| ix | INTRODUCTION | |
| **1** | **SECTION 1:** | **TERMINOLOGY AND IMPORTANT CONCEPTS** |
| 3 | CHAPTER 1: | Terminology |
| 13 | CHAPTER 2: | Concepts |
| **55** | **SECTION 2:** | **TEN REALMS OF BONDAGE** |
| 59 | CHAPTER 3: | Japanese Rope Bondage |
| 72 | | **TUTORIAL:** ***Single-Column Tie*** |
| 75 | | **TUTORIAL:** ***Double-Column Tie*** |
| 81 | CHAPTER 4: | Device Bondage |
| 96 | | **TUTORIAL:** ***Device Bondage Hogtie*** |
| 98 | | **TUTORIAL:** ***Crotch Rope*** |
| 102 | | **TUTORIAL:** ***Toothpick Heretic's Fork*** |
| 103 | CHAPTER 5: | Mental Bondage |
| 114 | | **TUTORIAL:** ***Position Training*** |
| 115 | | **TUTORIAL:** ***Mantra Training, a Precursor to Hypnosis*** |
| 117 | CHAPTER 6: | Objectification Bondage |
| 128 | | **TUTORIAL:** ***Balloon Bouncy Chair*** |
| 131 | | **TUTORIAL:** ***Pet Play Futomomo*** |
| 135 | CHAPTER 7: | Costume Bondage |
| 149 | | **TUTORIAL:** ***Master (Mistress, Mistrix)/ slave Collaring Ceremony*** |
| 149 | | **TUTORIAL:** ***Rope Body Harness*** |
| 154 | | **TUTORIAL:** ***DIY Hobble Skirt*** |
| 159 | CHAPTER 8: | Sensation Bondage |
| 170 | | **TUTORIAL:** ***Modifications for Pain*** |
| 170 | | **TUTORIAL:** ***Adult Swaddling*** |
| 174 | | **TUTORIAL:** ***Balloon Encasement*** |
| 179 | CHAPTER 9: | Fetish Bondage |
| 186 | | **TUTORIAL:** ***Foot Fetish: Nylon Encasement*** |

188 **TUTORIAL:** ***Sexy Clothing Bondage***

189 CHAPTER 10: Sensory Deprivation
203 **TUTORIAL:** ***Bedsheet and Belt Sleepsack***
206 **TUTORIAL:** ***Tape Hood with Nose Tubes***

209 CHAPTER 11: Physically Stressful Bondage
218 **TUTORIAL:** ***Predicament Tutorial***

219 CHAPTER 12: Self-Bondage
225 **TUTORIAL:** ***How to Make an Ice Lock***

**231 SECTION 3: EROTIC ESSAYS**

235 CHAPTER 13: Japanese Rope Bondage
*The God Particle* by Daemonumx

239 CHAPTER 14: Device Bondage
*Device of Destiny* by slave Destiny

243 CHAPTER 15: Mental Bondage
*Clarity and Devotion* by Domina Claire Hex, with consent from John

247 CHAPTER 16: Objectification Bondage
*Toy* by Domina Franco

253 CHAPTER 17: Costume Bondage
*Self-Discovery through Costume Bondage* by Mildred S. Pierce

257 CHAPTER 18: Sensation Bondage
*Sensation Overload: A Rebirth* by Mistress Couple

263 CHAPTER 19: Fetish Bondage
*Tension and Release* by Mistress Couple

269 CHAPTER 20: Sensory-Deprivation Bondage
*The Ultimate Supplication* by Mistress Tess NYC

273 CHAPTER 21: Predicament Bondage
*An Erotic and Fearsome Tale* by Karin Webb (aka Creature)

279 CHAPTER 22: Suspension Bondage
*Finding and Holding My Space* by Do

283 CHAPTER 23: Self-Bondage for One and Two
*Self-Bondage* by Master R

289 NOTES

293 ACKNOWLEDGMENTS

# INTRODUCTION

Welcome to *The Ultimate Guide to Bondage*! I'm Mistress Couple, and I am here to guide you on a journey into the complex and exciting world of erotic bondage. I'd like to tell you a little bit about myself so that you understand my background for writing this book. Like many, I arrived in the world of alternative sexuality through a long journey that involved many twists and turns. I've been kinky for my entire life, but it's hard to say when I first started intentionally seeking out bondage activities. A lot of my decision seems to stem back to my dance training.

Since the age of sixteen, I have studied ballroom and Latin dance techniques primarily, with some modern and ballet training mixed in. Learning how to control my body and make it move elegantly was a huge endeavor in mentally imposed discipline, and most likely my first erotic encounter with mental bondage. Taking my first steps in dance heels and pointe shoes was a humiliating foray into how debilitating different clothing or costume items could be. When I failed at producing the result that my dance coaches wanted to see (which was frequently), I'd be forced to dance with a broomstick bound to my back like a scarecrow to enforce good posture. Better yet, when my coach really wanted to torture me, I'd be placed in the predicament of trying to balance the broomstick across my arms as I demonstrated the proper ballroom dancing frame. I loved all of it. For me, the discipline, punishment, and pain were almost as delicious as the feeling of floating across the floor at the will of my partner. Yes, ballroom dancing even has elements of leading and following, dominance and submission.

In college, I continued my studies in dance, but also majored in psychology. I wanted to know not only what felt good in my body, but why it felt that way. I wanted to understand more about the human condition. Though my psychology classes provided a wonderful framework for understanding the science of the mind, bondage followed me to the dance department, and thus I focused most of my time there. One week into my freshman year, in a dance history course, an image of a woman stretching and straining within the confines of a Lycra garment shook me to the core. It was Martha Graham performing her famous ballet *Lamentation*. The emotion that she expressed, yearning to break through the boundaries that confined her, and bemoaning the bondage of the human condition, spoke to me on a deep, visceral level. Later that year I learned that the Graham company would be doing a summer residency at my school, and that I'd have the privilege of training with them and learning from them firsthand. I remember sitting on the floor of the dance studio with my back pressed against the glass, watching the company perform *Night Journey*, a ballet based on the Greek tragedy of *Oedipus Rex*.

The ballet starts at the moment Jocasta learns that she has mated with her own son, Oedipus, and borne him children. She dances with a piece of rope, twisting and contorting, and indicating that she wants to use the rope to end her life. The ballet then launches into a pas de deux between Jocasta and Oedipus that's intended to portray a flashback to a previous encounter between the two, using the rope as the primary prop. Throughout the ballet, Jocasta holds Oedipus as she would both a son and lover. In the end, the lovers wrap themselves in the rope, which has come to represent both the umbilical cord and the complicated tangle of their relationship.

Witnessing this dance was a formative moment in my understanding of bondage. Watching it for the first time, up close, I was riveted. The ballet was created in the late '40s and I found it hard to believe that such racy subject matter was addressed in plain sight! I also was astounded at Graham's brilliant use of such a simple prop. That night, I went to Home Depot and bought a piece of rope. I had to know, how did it feel to be wrapped up as the dancers in the ballet were?

Through a twist of fate that could only be characterized as luck, the curiosity sparked by Graham's *Night Journey* ended up guiding me to La Domaine Esemar, the oldest BDSM training château still in existence today. Before BDSM became mainstream and pop culture, there were small households similar to La Domaine scattered all over the world, where people could go to discreetly and privately be trained in the sadomasochistic arts. There, I was carefully ushered into the world of fetish exploration at the hands of Master R, Mistress Collette, and the rest of the La Domaine community, which they referred to as their family. Realizing that there was a great deal I could learn from these people, I offered myself to them as a slave. I wanted to give myself to them completely, and in return, to absorb as much training and insight as my brain and body could handle.

As it turned out, La Domaine was the perfect place to achieve what I had set out to do. Not just because of the expertise of Master R and Mistress Collette, but because of the vastly different perspectives and approaches I was exposed to at the hands of the other family members. La Domaine was not a place for judgment. Everyone was welcome, and every approach was considered to be valid, as long as the basic tenets of consent and safety were followed. Down in the La Domaine dungeon, I had the honor of being trained, bound, and even suspended by some of the best bondage Masters and Mistresses that the world had to offer.

Now, it is seven years later. Master R and Mistress Collette have both retired, and somehow, through the strange and complicated journey that life takes one on, I am no longer a slave, but the Head Mistress of the château. Now, it is my pleasure and responsibility to facilitate experiences similar to the ones that enlightened me. Having been on both sides of the rope gives me an amazing inventory of personal experiences to draw upon, and also provides some insight into my name.

Just as I switched between the roles of leader and follower on the ballroom dance floor, I now also switch roles in the dungeon. My submission informs my dominance, and vice versa. They are two parts of a whole. You know how ballroom dancers often wear numbers on their backs during competition? Thanks to Master R's astute sense of humor, my full name is actually "Couple Number 69." That might be more than you'd ever care to know about me.

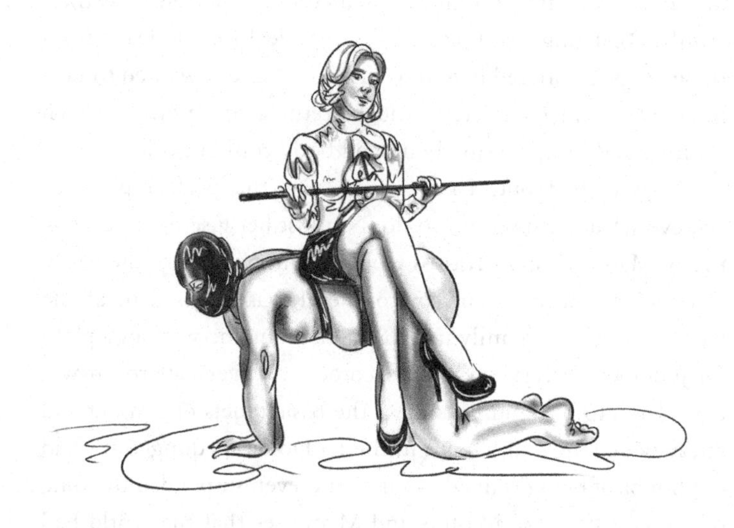

## OK, enough about you . . . what about the book?

Now that we are acquainted, I'll continue by letting you know: This book aims to be different than your standard Rope 101 book (if you hadn't yet gathered that by my introduction!). If you picked up this book in hopes of learning to tie rope, well, you'll find plenty on that topic embedded within (see our chapter on Japanese rope bondage). However, the aim of this book is to be much more expansive and encompassing in addressing bondage in its totality.

This book aims to guide you on a journey into all realms of bondage, as I endeavor to demonstrate that there is so very much more to the topic than simply rope! From mechanical devices, to costume bondage, to bondage that aims to go beyond simple restraint and engages the participants' deep intentional connection, there is a lot for us to explore together. By drawing references from both culture and history, I'll demonstrate that bondage extends far beyond the underground BDSM scene and often is hiding in plain sight!

It is my deepest hope that there is something for everyone to learn from this book. Whether you are nervously dipping your toes into the world of alternative sexuality for the first time or are an experienced bondage practitioner, there are insights and suggestions in this book that should help you to expand your perception of what bondage is.

Borrowing a stylistic choice from my favorite BDSM text, *Sacred Kink* by Lee Harrington, each chapter will include sections to address different areas of interest.[1] For the philosophers and psychologically inclined, I have put forth a lot of unique new insights, connecting my personal knowledge of psychology, professional domination, and bondage. For the academics and history buffs, there's a great deal of material to dive into about

---

1 Lee Harrington, *Sacred Kink* (Lynwood: Mystic Productions LLC, 2009).

the origins of different forms of bondage. The hands-on learners will read about how to select the appropriate tools for a bondage scenario and will be able to put their skills to the test by engaging in the tutorials in each chapter. Most of the tutorials include materials that are household items or can be easily sourced, so you don't have to wait to get started! Best of all, included at the end of the book are a number of firsthand accounts intended to vicariously transport you into the bondage experiences you just learned about. In order to provide a variety of voices and perspectives for you to consider, many of these essays have been written by bondage mentors, victims, and friends I have had the pleasure of exploring with at La Domaine Esemar.

Before you get to all that good stuff, you'll need to start out in Section 1. Section 1 includes terminology and important concepts to consider and is meant to serve as an orientation. Think of this section as a key to the map of the terrain that we will explore together. If you're new to this world, you'll definitely want to read these chapters, otherwise you might find yourself lost. If you're already well versed in BDSM 101, I'd still suggest skimming through, as you might find a new perspective or tool to add to your bag of tricks. There's also a large section on safety protocols that you'll want to read to jog your memory.

Many of the topics in Section 1 are probably a lot heavier than you'd expect for the tone of a how-to book, but it is important to me that you understand that bondage isn't all fun and games and sex. Yes, it can be that, and I hope that by the end of the book, you are able to enjoy it as such. However, it is also my hope that you are able to engage in it with ideal intent, by understanding the gravity of the endeavor you're about to embark on and how bondage affects the human condition. Section 1 will do its best to convey this to you.

In Section 2, we'll take a journey into ten different realms of bondage: Japanese rope bondage, device bondage, mental bondage, objectification bondage, costume bondage, sensation bondage, fetish bondage, sensory-deprivation bondage, physically stressful bondage, and self-bondage. There is a flow chart that you can use at the end of Section 1, which, based on your answers, will guide you to the chapter in Section 2 that suits your interests or personality the most. If you don't know where to start, you're the choose-your-own-adventure type, or you simply cannot wait to dive into your favorite bondage topic, the flow chart will serve as an effective shortcut. That being said, the ten chapters in Section 2 are structured in the order that seems like the most logical path to me, and build off one another in a way that is intended to provide some sort of method to the madness.

What madness, you ask? For the purposes of organization, it was necessary to label the bondage activities and section them off into different categories. Continuing with our map metaphor, you can think of them as small stops along a train line, each stop leading to a specific destination in terms of end result. In reality, though, bondage activities are not so easy to reduce into bite-size pieces. Oftentimes a single BDSM interaction will include multiple realms of bondage, fused together like the cars of a train. In these types of interactions, there's really no saying where you'll end up once you leave the station. Your final destination will be determined by the conductor (giving partner), passengers (receiving partners), weather conditions (mental state of partners), traffic conditions (trauma histories), and a variety of other factors. You'll be able to see examples of how the different bondage realms meld together in the essays in Section 3. Hopefully, these stories will inspire you to mix and match the skills that you learn in each of the separate realms as you so desire.

Section 4 will provide a completely new map, to guide you on your next exploration into the world of bondage.

In addition to an educational adventure, this is intended to be a guided self-exploration. Throughout the book, you will find a recurring theme: the revelation of things that were once hidden or buried deep within the soul. Sometimes, these revelations can be joyous, at other times they can be challenging to process, so I urge you to breathe deeply, proceed slowly, and allow yourself time to process each section. After all, you picked up this book to learn about bondage, and what better way is there to do that than to liberate your own thoughts? Are you ready? Here we go. Prepare yourself for a journey into the complex world of erotic bondage.

SECTION 1:

# TERMINOLOGY AND IMPORTANT CONCEPTS

CHAPTER 1

# TERMINOLOGY

It is important, before we embark on this journey together, to know that we are speaking the same language—both linguistically and conceptually. Here you will find a glossary of terminology that is crucial to exploring the bondage community, and important to know so that we can communicate effectively.

## General Terms

**Vanilla:** Vanilla is a term that is used within alternative communities to refer to activities, specifically of the sexual kind, which are socially deemed normal. The term is also used to refer to so-called normal scenarios, such as spending time with family members, working in a profession, or being in public.

**Kinky:** Kinky is a term that refers to sexual behaviors that fall outside the socially deemed category of normal. But of course, there is no one way in which to be normal. Each person's normal is different! That's what being kinky is all about: going against the grain and embracing parts of your sexuality that are unique. Kink activities can be associated with intercourse-based sex, but they frequently do not venture into the territory of intercourse at all. As opposed to an orgasm, in kinky activities, the experiences of connection, control, and sensation are often seen as end goals. For those who do not experience arousal, it is also possible to engage in kinky activities without a sexual context, with the same end goals in mind. Kinky activities can include bondage, role play, fetish and fantasy exploration, and other alternative expressions of personhood.

**Scene:** A scene is where two or more people come together to engage in kinky activities. A scene can refer to a specific occurrence between two people (i.e., "We did a spanking scene together") or to the community at large ("Are you in the BDSM scene?").

**Play:** *Play* is a word that is used to refer to the practice of BDSM activities (i.e., "Do you want to play?"). *Play partner* is used to describe someone with whom you engage in BDSM activities regularly.

**Munch:** A munch is a get-together of kinky people at a public location such as a diner or bar. It gives people the opportunity to meet other kinksters and vet potential partners in a safe environment.

**Edge play:** Edge play is the thrill seeker's play preference. It involves pushing boundaries, exploring something challenging, and walking right up to the edge of your personal limits. Typically, edge play involves much more risk than the typical tie-and-tease. Play involving fire, blood, or the potential for psychological or mental damage are often considered to be edge play. A more literal type of edge play involves playing with sharp edges such as knives or other cutting implements. Keeping all of that in mind, edge play is determined entirely by who is playing, since what feels threatening to one person might seem boring to another. It is about finding where your limits are so that you can work to transcend them.

## Power Exchange and BDSM

The world runs on power dynamics. They are embedded at every level of our society and are fundamental to how we interact with one another, consensually or not. In our day-to-day lives, factors that *shouldn't* be at play—factors such as race, age, gender, sex, disability, education, and wealth distribution—have tragically come to dictate these dynamics.

In BDSM, we aim to rebuild them on our own terms—coming from a place of awareness of these power structures. We aim to create structures of dominance and submission that are not built upon these societal factors, but that start and end with desire and consent.

That said, this is all but impossible in our society without an awareness of structures that are already in place. Power dynamics are a loaded topic. Trying to enter into a consensual power-exchange dynamic, wherein a partner voluntarily assumes or relinquishes control, can be very difficult without first addressing the position of power or powerlessness you come from within the context of society as a whole.

If you are white, if you are a man, if you come from a position of wealth, whether you are cognizant of it or not, our society elevates your privilege. It is important to be aware of this, and to check these things as you start to explore consensual power exchange. This process is also sometimes referred to as examining your privilege and will be covered more in the next chapter.

Power-exchange dynamics do not always denote inequality. In many vanilla relationships, partners negotiate who does the laundry and who pays the bills. Some people feel more comfortable in a 1950s housewife-type role where their partner is the breadwinner and therefore holds more power in the relationship; others prefer more equality in a partnership. As long as the power dynamics within a relationship are put in place with the blessing of both partners, society as a whole considers those relationships to be healthy. In consensual erotic power-exchange dynamics, the same sort of negotiation happens, but is focused more on roles of power within the bedroom or sexual encounters. Beyond the typical negotiation of what sexual positions you want to use or who gets to be "on top" (a position of control) during sex, folks who engage in erotic power-exchange dynamics take a lot of time parsing out their desires in terms of control or lack of control in sexual scenarios. Usually, these desires involve the negotiation of BDSM activities.

**BDSM** is a term that is intended to cover the following activities:
**B&D or B/D:** Bondage and discipline
**D&S or D/s:** Dominance and submission
**S&M or SM:** Sadism and masochism
**SM** is also used in reference to "sex magick."

Many books have been written on all of these topics; as this book focuses on bondage, let us take a moment to explore what exactly that word means.

**Bondage:** According to the *Merriam-Webster Collegiate Dictionary*,[2] there are three definitions of the word *bondage*.

1: tenure or service of a villein, serf, or slave.
2: a state of being bound usually by compulsion (as of law or mastery): such as
 a: captivity, serfdom
 b: servitude or subjugation to a controlling person or force
3: sadomasochistic sexual practices involving the physical restraint of one partner.

These first two definitions allude to bondage as something other than the kinky sex fantasies that come to mind when most of us hear the word in modern vernacular. Though we explore it today as a consensual leisure activity, it is important to bear in mind that bondage has a sordid and dark history of nonconsensual imprisonment, and as with power exchange, this is something important to unpack and be cognizant of on our journey.

Many of today's consensual bondage activities are evolved from skills that were originally intended to impose involuntary slavery and torture. The reappropriation and reclamation of these same activities into tools for creating closeness, for building bonds between partners, is a demonstration of democracy in action. Through the application of principles like consent, safewords, and aftercare (which you'll learn about in the next chapter), bondage can be transformed into a safe, enjoyable activity for participants to choose to engage in.

While on the topic of the definition of bondage: You might think of bondage primarily as a way to keep people from moving, but it is so much more than that.

---

2 *Merriam-Webster*, s.v. "Bondage (n.)," accessed October 4, 2017, https://www.merriam-webster.com/dictionary/bondage.

To start with, physical restraint is not the only meaningful way to hold someone captive: Mental bondage, costume bondage, objectification, sensory deprivation, etc., can all be mechanisms of restraint and control. Yes, part of bondage is about creating restrictions, but the other part of it is about creating sensations on a spectrum ranging from ethereal sensual floating to sadistic pain. If you were worried that bondage might not be for you because it's too "forceful," think again! It can actually be quite gentle and nurturing.

**Discipline:** The *D* in BDSM has multiple meanings; the first of these is discipline. In this context, discipline is the practice of teaching your partner to obey your commands, or to follow the rules that you set. In this sense, discipline is a form of mental restraint—whether the restraint is caused by a fear of punishment or a desire to please, your partner becomes bound by your will.

In most instances, the binding agent is the former: Discipline tends to mean the use of punishment (physical or otherwise) to correct disobedience. This is inherent in the origins of modern-day BDSM; our roots stem from the gay leather scene that was developed in the 1940s by military veterans.[3] In a military organization, (semi-)consensual power dynamics become a codified way of life, as do the forms of discipline and punishment used to enforce them. These were the seeds from which our movement initially grew.

We all have consensual and nonconsensual experiences with discipline and power. When we slave to the traffic light, obediently waiting out a red light in spite of the absence of cross traffic, that is discipline at work. We may prefer to put the pedal to the metal, but our fear of a punishing ticket or unpleasant encounter

---

3 GLBTQ Encyclopedia (archive), "Leather Culture," by Matthew D. Johnson, accessed June 13, 2018, http://www.glbtqarchive.com/ssh/leather_culture_S.pdf.

with law enforcement restrains us. We often discipline ourselves to work or study for fear of being fired from our jobs or receiving bad grades. Plenty of people have received discipline from their parents in the form of a spanking or being grounded. In erotic contexts, discipline takes on a different form. It is used as a way to enforce control over a sexual situation, and to mold someone into the ideal sexual partner. In many cases, people who engage in consensual BDSM activities enjoy being disciplined. With that in mind, it is also important to acknowledge that because of the trauma-producing nature of nonconsensual discipline, exploring this concept can be very difficult for people who have a history that involves it, and thus it should be handled delicately.

**Dominance:** In my opinion, society has a very confused understanding of the qualities that indicate erotic dominance. Typically, a dominant person is seen as loud, brash, or "large and in charge." That is not dominant; it is domineering. To me, being dominant means being a good leader, and thus contains elements of empathy, respect, and self-awareness. Within the BDSM community, the word *Dominant* (Dom or Domme for short) is used to refer to people who assume the role of power and control within an ongoing power exchange relationship. Other titles for Dominant partners are Mistress (feminine), Master (masculine), or Mistrix (gender neutral). The title is typically capitalized to denote that role of power (whereas the word *submissive* is typically lowercase). Those who use a dominant title usually think of themselves as enforcing a constant hierarchy in the relationship. Those who only want to engage in power exchange occasionally, or desire a more casual dynamic between play partners, generally use the title of Top.

**Submission:** It is also my opinion that society misconstrues erotic submission. Like with most misconceptions about BDSM, the distinction has to do with consent. Whereas in nonconsensual settings, the act of submission stems from a place of powerlessness or weakness, voluntary submission requires a great deal of strength, both physical and of character. Voluntary submission requires the maturity and self-awareness to recognize the beauty in giving power as a gift to those you deem most worthy of it. As the house motto of La Domaine Esemar states, "It's not about how much you can take, but how much you can give." Many people who identify as full-time erotic submissives choose to use the title of "slave." It is important to acknowledge the fact that the word *slave* has different connotations based on one's level of privilege, and therefore it should only be used as a title for those who make a conscious decision to use it.

For example, as someone with nonconsensual slavery in my family history, I found it to be very empowering to reclaim the word *slave* as a part of my identity. Within the context of a consensual Master/slave dynamic, it helped me to examine the submissive parts of my personality and realize who deserves my submission and devotion and who does not. That being said, I acknowledge my privilege as a white-passing woman, and understand that the implications of slavery are not the same for me as a Jewish woman as they might be for an African American, or someone with a history of nonconsensual sex trafficking.

If you'd prefer to avoid using the loaded term *slave*, other titles include "sub," "submissive," "bottom," or "pet." Of course, you're always welcome to make one up that you feel suits you better than these terms, and I encourage you to do so.

**Top/bottom/switch:** Within the context of a scene, the top is the person who is in charge. It is the top's role to initiate activities and physically act upon the bottom. The bottom is the receiver of the action and attention. Topping and bottoming does not necessarily denote a power dynamic between partners; in fact, tops and bottoms typically view themselves to be on an equal playing field within the context of control of the scene. Whereas "topping from the bottom," or trying to control the experience, is frowned upon in power-exchange dynamics, it is viewed as appropriate when there is no power dynamic between partners. Think of it as guiding your masseuse to the spot that needs the most work, or teaching a new lover about the sensations that your body finds to be pleasurable. Take note, though—if you're a bottom who is constantly telling your top exactly what to do, you might be a switch, or someone who is inclined toward both roles. Whether someone becomes a top or bottom can change based on a variety of factors including their mood, the partner they're playing with, or the activity that they are engaging in. Some even people switch roles midscene!

**Sadism/masochism:** Sadism and masochism will be addressed in greater detail throughout the book, but for now it is important that you understand that they are words that refer to different causes of arousal. Sadism refers to arousal that is experienced through inflicting pain on someone or watching them be hurt, whereas masochism connotes arousal from experiencing pain. The terms can be used to refer to either physical or emotional pain.

**Subspace/Top-space:** The cocktail of chemical neurotransmitters and hormones such as oxytocin, adrenaline, and endorphins that are released in response to BDSM play can cause altered states of mental processing.[4] It is difficult to pin down what these headspaces actually entail, as they're different for everyone depending on a variety of factors, but there are some unifying

4 Ossiana Tepfenhart, "This Is What BDSM Does to Your Brain According to Science," *Rebel Circus* (blog), October 5, 2016, http://www.rebelcircus.com/blog/bdsm-brain-according-science/.

characteristics among people's reports. Whereas subspace reportedly feels relaxed, floaty, and even sometimes quite disoriented/inebriated, top-space is often referred to as "supercharged," and is accompanied by an overactive mind. Both states of mind are highly sought after by those who engage in BDSM practices, but are approached with the same caution and respect as one would approach other mind-altering substances.

**Sex magic(k):** Any type of sexual activity that is used in magical, ritualistic, religious, and spiritual endeavors falls under the umbrella of sex magic(k). The use of the letter *k* was coined by Aleister Crowley (founder of Thelemic mysticism) to denote a difference between the occult and performance magic. Many sex magick practitioners believe that their bodies are able to transcend physical realities and connect to the universe by engaging in sexual intercourse.[5] One of the most widely practiced aspects of sex magic involves visualization of a desired outcome during orgasm.[6] Sex magick is commonly associated with BDSM play, not just because the two are often used in conjunction with one another, but also because through deep examination of our relationships to bondage, discipline, dominance, submission, sadism, and masochism, our perceptions of society and reality are transformed.

**Rigger:** Rigger is a term that is commonly used within the bondage community to refer to an experienced bondage top. Typically, riggers are people who use rope as their primary bondage tool, and people who have a high level of competency in regards to rope suspension.

---

5 Charlotte Szivak, "Sex Magic Alchemy," *Medium* (blog), December 16, 2013, https://medium.com/the-divine-o/sex-magic-alchemy-5042d22289c5.

6 Damon Brand, *Adventures in Sex Magick: Control Your Life With the Power of Lust* (The Gallery of Magick, 2014), 5.

CHAPTER

# 2

# CONCEPTS

Now that you are equipped with the knowledge of commonly used bondage terminology, let's take a look at some concepts that will lead you farther down the path of discovery and closer to achieving your bondage goals.

## Privilege

Although we touched on this concept a bit while discussing power exchange, I think that it is important to delve deeper into it. Talking about privilege tends to get our backs up and put us on the defensive because of feelings of guilt or the desire to avoid blame. This does nothing to help society progress, and in fact, our own refusal to accept blame sets us back. Realizing that privilege is not always directly caused by our actions, but by the complicity of society as a whole, is an important step toward liberation, and thus I'd like to offer some more thoughts on the topic.

San Francisco educator and activist Sam Dylan Finch raises the following questions regarding what privilege means:

Does having privilege mean that you do not struggle or suffer?

Does having privilege mean that you are a bad person?

The answer to both is no. He follows with this excellent comment about his own privilege: "It simply means that I gained an unearned advantage, in comparison to other people—by no fault of my own, but rather, because of prejudice."

He further explains that, "When someone asks you to 'check your privilege,' what they're really asking you to do is to reflect on the ways that your social status might have given you an advantage—*even if you didn't ask for it or earn it*—while their social status might have given them a disadvantage."[7]

If you are choosing to engage in erotic bondage, it is because you have the privilege to do so. It is important to take note that even as you are reading right now, there are folks in this world who are being subjected to bondage in a nonconsensual manner. There are folks who have been incarcerated or have been affected by the incarceration of a family member. There are folks who have a history of nonconsensual bondage in their lineage. Instances where nonconsensual power dynamics are imposed on people are generally considered to be traumatic and often cause long-term effects such as post-traumatic stress disorder (PTSD), panic attacks, stress, and anxiety. References to power exchange, consensual or not, might dredge up (or trigger) and exacerbate these conditions. The last thing that you want to do during sexy time is cause unintended emotional distress for your partner, so it is important to be mindful of their history.

Even if someone has not experienced trauma directly, scientific evidence shows that stress disorders can be passed down

---

7 Sam Dylan Finch, "Ever Been Told to 'Check Your Privilege?' Here's What That Really Means," *Everyday Feminism* (blog), July 27, 2015, https://everydayfeminism.com/2015/07/what-checking-privilege-means/.

through DNA.[8] Therefore, if someone has a family history of trauma or nonconsensual power exchange, they are likely to be triggered, similarly to (although typically not as intensely as) someone who experienced a traumatic event during their lifetime. Because this is a fairly recent scientific discovery, many people are confused by their adverse reactions to witnessing consensual BDSM play. Make sure that you thoroughly examine your own trauma history and discuss your partners' with them, too. Be considerate about the position of power (or powerlessness) from which you approach erotic bondage. You are lucky to have the privilege of freedom to explore this topic, and you should not abuse it.

## Ethics

Societal views of what values and principles are deemed morally right or wrong are constantly evolving. This is especially true in the world of BDSM, where there is not one unified ethical guideline, but different codes of ethics that morph to meet unique spaces and situations; what makes sense in your private bedroom may not translate to a public party or workshop. Despite this lack of unifying law, there are some important underlying principles for conducting oneself during a bondage scene that will help to keep everyone happy and coming back for more sexy fun time! When engaging in a practice such as bondage, it's not enough to simply say that you are an ethical person—you must act in accordance with those ethics. In the age of the internet, bondage enthusiasts have formed a virtual network and often ban unethical players from workshops and events. Baseline: Don't be a jerk! Be humble, too. When you engage in BDSM activities, you

---

8 Tori Rodriguez. "Descendants of Holocaust Survivors Have Altered Stress Hormones," *Scientific American*, March 1, 2015, https://www.scientificamerican.com/article/descendants-of-holocaust-survivors-have-altered-stress-hormones/.

are placing your life in someone else's hands, or taking their life into yours. If you respect your partner's life, want to behave ethically, and want to try to avoid causing a traumatic event (with the understanding that mistakes do happen), continue reading this chapter and make a pact with yourself to adhere to these guidelines. It will save you and your partners a lot of grief in the future.

## Consent

The fundamental building block for any relationship or sexual encounter is consent. Securing informed consent from your partner is imperative, whether it is a first encounter or fiftieth-anniversary romp. Never assume that you know what someone else wants to have done to or with their body, as our bodies and states of mind are constantly in flux. Based on the context of our daily lives, being gagged could feel very relaxing on one day and incredibly frustrating the next. The act of erotic bondage inherently creates a power dynamic and deep sense of vulnerability between practitioners, therefore, asking for and receiving consent is an important first step in the trust building that needs to occur each time that you play.

When asking for consent, you need to make sure that you clearly express what activities you are asking your partner to engage in. Make sure that you get an enthusiastic YES! from anyone that you ask to participate. When giving consent, make sure that you are fully informed of the risks that are involved in the proposed activity (pay attention—there will be more information about risk aversion and safety in each chapter, as there are different risks associated with different types of bondage). Make sure that you've discussed what's expected to happen, shared concerns that you have, talked about your limits, and then, and only then, enthusiastically agreed to participate. When you ask for or give consent, you should do so willingly, without pressure, coercion, or reservation. It's important to note that asking for consent from someone who is under the influence of drugs or alcohol is considered to be coercion and should be avoided. Avoiding drugs and alcohol when engaging in bondage is a good general rule, as you will want to be as sharp and alert as possible so that you're able to communicate effectively.

### *Consent Challenges for Bottoms*

**Speak up!** Oftentimes, new bottoms are worried to use their safeword because they're afraid that ending the scene will disappoint their partner. It is important to keep in mind that it would be far more disappointing for the Top to find out that they injured or hurt their bottom unintentionally. There are so many fun bondage activities that exist in the world—it does no good to take someone (including yourself) to a place they're not ready to visit yet. If you find yourself struggling from mental or physical strain during a scene, or even if you're just not feeling it, say something IMMEDIATELY. Communicate with your partner using the systems that are discussed later in this chapter. Voicing discomfort doesn't necessitate the end of a scene; on the contrary, it can support the longevity of one.

### *Consent Challenges for Tops*

**Be responsible!** As a bondage Top, you're going to be responsible for the well-being of your partner. Make sure that you're aware of all the risks involved in the activity that you'd like to explore, and be prepared in the case of an emergency.

With new play partners, especially those who are new to sexual exploration, it is advisable to operate on the principle of not trusting someone's yes until they give you a no. In other words, do not go charging ahead unless you are positive that your partner can effectively assert their boundaries and limits. The negotiation process will assist with this.

### *What happens if a limit is crossed?*

We are all human and we are all capable of making mistakes, but there is a BIG difference between accidentally violating consent and intentionally violating consent. Whereas intentional consent violations occur when someone deliberately ignores or crosses a partner's limits, consent accidents happen because of misjudgments, miscommunications, faulty assumptions, or not having all the pertinent details about your play partner. If a limit is crossed, even accidentally, it might be upsetting, and in some cases traumatic. This can make determining whether a breach of consent was intentional or accidental very difficult. As such, it can be incredibly hard for the victim of a consent violation to address the perpetrator, so if you are the partner who crossed a limit, being proactive about your transgression is important.

**If you were the person to accidentally cause the breach of consent:** Taking accountability for your actions and working to address your behavior is imperative. Apologizing for your partner's pain, without problem solving or blaming, is a good first step. A simple "I'm so sorry that you got hurt" will suffice.

Empathizing with your partner will allow them to see that you truly feel sorry for hurting them, and stating that you did not intend to hurt them is also helpful. After acknowledging your partner's pain, you can look more closely at the details. You didn't mean to hurt them, but it still happened—why? Maybe there was a miscommunication during your initial negotiation, and you misunderstood what your partner was asking for in the play scenario. Maybe they said their safeword, but you were playing in a loud club and didn't hear it. Identify the source of the mistake, acknowledge it, and apologize for it. This is a different apology than the first, as it should contain details that show your partner that you now truly understand how the accidental breach happened, and you take responsibility for it.

Tell your partner what you'll do to prevent making the mistake in the future. In many cases, you can learn from the mistake you've made and use it to improve your play dynamics and communication skills. Having a plan to avert such accidents in future scenarios will also go a long way toward rebuilding trust.

Finally, ask your partner if they have any other needs that don't feel met. Based on how upsetting the consent breach was to them, they might need some time apart to figure out what they need. Give it to them. Set up a time to check in, or let them be in control about when to resume contact. In the meantime, don't beat yourself up. Rather, acknowledge that there are many reasons we might accidentally hurt someone, and examine what you could do to better yourself.

**If you were the person whose limits were crossed:** If the violation was minor, you might be able to address your limits in the moment. Do so loudly and assertively. If the violation was serious, or caused physical or emotional harm or trauma, you will most likely not be able to address it immediately. Make it clear that a boundary has been crossed and you're upset, and find a way to leave. If it was an intentional breach of consent, such as a rape or sexual assault, it's advisable that you report the situation and seek medical attention. If you do not feel comfortable doing so, that's okay. Sexual assault scenarios are vastly different and uniquely challenging for each victim, and everyone has the right to handle their assault in the way they choose. For the purposes of this section, we will focus on accidental or unintentional consent violations.

While you're processing a breach of consent, identifying where things went wrong can be very difficult. Give yourself some space and time to "come down" from the stress of the experience before trying to identify whether it was intentional or an accident. Check in with yourself about your fear response system. Was your instinct to fight, fly, flee, or freeze? How did that play into the scenario? Once you are ready, you may want to seek out support from a friend, trauma counselor, or therapist to help you sort out what happened. If you determine that the violation was an accident and choose to have a discussion with your partner, do so with a full understanding of what your limits were, what went wrong, and what you'd like to be done in order to avoid repeats in the future. Remember, you are never obligated to give feedback to someone if you aren't comfortable doing so.

Taking action and participating in these steps will do a lot to reduce resentment between partners in accidental scenarios. Educating yourself about how to handle consent breaches in case something happens will allow you to enter into a tense situation prepared, rather than with your guard up. All that being said, starting off with a solid negotiation process will lessen the chances of miscommunication in the first place. Keep reading to learn how to thoroughly and fairly negotiate a BDSM scenario.[9]

## Negotiation

Negotiation is a term used to refer to discussions that play out before a scene, to discern where participants' interests, desires, comfort levels, and boundaries lie for whatever activities may be on the table.

With a new partner, it is strongly advised to be both thorough and systematic in negotiation. This approach ensures that all the bases are covered—that everything that could come into play in the scene is discussed beforehand, and the boundaries of

---

9 Charlie Glickman, "Consent Accidents and Consent Violations," *Make Sex Easy* (blog), http://www.makesexeasy.com/consent-accidents-consent-violations/.

consent are very clear. Moreover, a thorough negotiation gives participants in a scene more of an opportunity to understand and empathize with each other beforehand, which can be very helpful in facilitating in-scene connection.

Some topics to consider include: What power dynamics and roles do you want to explore? Topping and bottoming? Dominance and submission? Sadism and masochism? What kinds of sensations are sought and consented to? Sensual? Painful? Sexual? If sexual play is on the table, what does that look like for both partners? What kinds of protection are necessary? What body parts do you and your partner consent to be interacted with, and in what ways? With what intent? Are toys going to be used? What toys? Are there role plays that you and your partner want to explore? What do those look like? Where do interest, desire, willingness, and consent stand for each of these things? Etc. . . .

An important topic to keep in mind while negotiating is your "risk budget." That is to say, no activity—in kink, sex, or life itself—is entirely predictable or free of risk. It is important to keep this in mind when negotiating: to know the potential risks of anything you consent to, and only give consent to that which falls within your budget of risk.

Special care must be given to so-called edge play topics—those with the most obvious danger to do damage if not handled carefully. Consensual nonconsent, or CNC, is one such topic requiring especially large amounts of care. This is where one partner—usually a bottom/submissive—consents to their partner pushing them beyond their usual boundaries, into territory to which they would not otherwise have consented. It is imperative, if exploring this, to fully discuss what this means for each party involved, if safewords are required, if there are areas that are off-limits even within the CNC paradigm, etc. This is advanced-level consent requiring advanced-level negotiations, and should only be approached with extreme caution.

It's easy to miss topics in negotiation; to help avoid this, some people come into negotiations with a checklist, or form, to work off. This can include a plethora of different fetishes, power dynamics, sexual activities, body parts, etc. Working from a form, wherein each participant can rank their interest/ desire (from zero to ten) for any given item, and level of consent (yes/no/ask first/etc.) for said activity, can be a good model to operate from.

It is important to keep in mind that, as a dynamic evolves, changes, and shifts, so do the consent models at play. Frequently, as partners become more comfortable with each other, certain areas require renegotiation—for instance, an activity that was out-of-bounds may now be open to explore, or other areas may no longer be welcome. Therefore, it's imperative that negotiations occur regularly and frequently throughout a relationship.

As dynamics evolve, negotiations often trend toward becoming looser and less formal. As partners get to know each other better, often they will even choose to negotiate out long-standing consent models, sometimes foregoing prescene negotiation altogether. An extreme example might be that of "passive consent," wherein one partner consents to any and all activity on the part of their partner, except for prenegotiated hard limits or no-fly zones. However, this is only acceptable as a conscious choice that all participants have made of their own accord; if that hasn't been reached and discussed, sticking with formal, thorough negotiations is incredibly important for maintaining consensual, safe play.

Once negotiations have been settled, and a scene has started, it's important that all participants share responsibility to keep the scene within the negotiated boundaries. Failing to do so, and choosing to negotiate on the fly midscene—when endorphins are flowing, headspaces are altered, power dynamics are in place, etc.—can lead to reckless decisions and is not advisable. If a new, hot idea occurs to you midscene, and you are not 100 percent certain that it falls within negotiated territory that your partner has already consented to, save it for next time.

## Safety and Responsibility

I wish that I could tell you that engaging in bondage activities is completely safe, but that would not be true. Do plenty of people engage in bondage activities all the time without getting hurt? Yes, but those people practice a great deal of risk analysis and aversion; in other words, they know what they're doing. Honestly, even the most skilled bondage practitioners have things go wrong sometimes. We're all human, after all, and we're subject to making errors in judgment or practice. It's pretty common sense that if you're unaware of the risks associated with an activity, you're more likely to accidentally do something dangerous. I've heard plenty of stories of childhood self-bondage experiments from friends (and participated in some myself) that to this day make me cringe! As your guide, it's my job to inform you of the importance of bondage safety, so allow me to spell this out for you very clearly:

PARTICIPATING IN BONDAGE IS NEVER RISK-FREE.

Whether you are planning on Topping or bottoming, if you're engaging in bondage activities, it's imperative that you understand the risks involved. Risk assessment is a tricky topic because everybody's physicality, psyche, skill level, and relationship dynamics are different. That means that there are different risks involved for each individual every time they enter a new scenario or play with a different partner. It's highly recommended that you engage in a thorough negotiation process before each and every bondage experience that you engage in. There are a few bondage-safety concepts that apply to everyone, regardless of individual differences, and these concepts should be considered with the utmost regard and respect.

WHEN YOU ENGAGE IN BONDAGE,
SOMEONE'S LIFE IS ON THE LINE.
SO PAY ATTENTION.

### *Safety Tools*

**Safety shears:** In the case of an emergency, you're going to have to be able to remove someone from bondage as quickly as possible. Safety shears are typically used by paramedics and have a rounded bulb rather than a blade on the bottom so that they can slide underneath clothing or other material and cut it without the risk of cutting the flesh. MAKE SURE THAT YOUR SAFETY SHEARS CAN CUT THROUGH WHATEVER BONDAGE MATERIAL YOU'RE USING *BEFORE* YOU USE IT. Get to know how your tool works, and have it on hand rather than across the room so that in an emergency situation, you can respond quickly and without struggle.

**Bolt cutters:** For metal bondage devices such as chains and locks, safety shears aren't going to do the trick. If you want to save yourself the embarrassment of having to call the fire department or drive to Home Depot while bound, it's best to have a pair of these around.

**First-aid kit:** Have a first-aid kit on hand and know how to provide aid for the risks associated with your play.

**Water bottle:** A water bottle with a squeeze top, a bottle, or a sippy cup are important to have on hand in case your partner is dehydrated or light-headed and bound. This way, you can help them hydrate without having to wait to release all of the bondage devices.

**Hard point:** A hard point is a fixed point that you tie bondage off to, such as a bedpost, support beam, bolted eye hook, or ring. It is important to make sure that your hard point is secure and load tested for weight.

### *Physical Risks*[10]

**Circulation impairment:** While blood restriction is sometimes the goal of bondage play, if neglected, it can be too much of a good thing (in the Shakespearean sense of the term—ouch!). When left for too long, hypoxia sets in on the tied-off limb, ushering in a number of potential complications, including but not limited to blood clots or gangrene. If a limb is denied good circulation for long enough, it's possible that it would have to be amputated. So if you want to keep your parts intact, pay attention!

Mindfulness around materials used and the placement and pressure of those materials should aid in mitigating risk for reduced circulation. The most important factor for determining pressure is the amount of material that is against the skin. This is especially true in cases where the bondage will be load bearing or the bottom will be pulling against the restraints. The more coverage the bondage device has, the more dispersed the pressure against the bonds will be, and the more comfortable the bottom will be. With rope or other wrapping mediums, the number of wraps around the limb determines thickness. Most riggers like to use at least an inch of coverage (two to five wraps depending on

---

10 Pete Riggs, "The Safety Series Part 1: Physical Risk with Rope Bondage," *Rope Connections* (blog), July 31, 2015, https://www.ropeconnections.com/the-safety-series-part-1-physical-risk-with-rope-bondage/. Shay Tiziano and Stefanos Tiziano, "Introduction and Basic Risks," *Remedial Ropes* (blog), http://www.remedialropes.com/basic-bondage-safety/introduction-and-basic-risks/.

the rope that you're using) for tying up limbs. Using more wraps for larger-bodied or sensitive partners and fewer wraps for pain-seeking partners are modifications that you can use to create a personalized rope experience.

When considering which materials to use, bear in mind that highly stretchy materials, such as bungee cords, nylon stockings, balloons, and rubber bands, can act like a tourniquet.[11] When using these materials, be extra careful about circulatory issues. Softer bondage materials with less pliability (leather, rope, silk scarves, handkerchiefs, etc.) are less likely to cause problems but still have the potential to do so, so remain vigilant.

Other considerations for placement and pressure include avoiding vulnerable areas with little fat or muscle (such as joints) and leaving some wiggle room for blood flow. Follow the two-finger rule by leaving your wraps loose enough to slide two fingers underneath. Do not mistake tightness for security. If you are using the correct techniques, it is possible to leave devices loose enough that they reduce risk and tight enough that your partner cannot escape.

Once bound, if you feel any tingling, numbness, throbbing, stinging, or pain in the limb that is tied off, immediately adjust or even completely remove the bondage device. A little change in coloration of the limb is to be expected, but if the limb begins to turn blue or white, that is a signal that oxygen levels in the blood are low. Variation in skin tone can make it difficult to assess what determines dangerous levels of discoloration, so it is advisable to pay more heed to changes in skin temperature (cooling is an indication of danger) and comfort levels. That being said, use common sense and always err on the side of caution. If a limb is cold, very discolored, or doesn't have a pulse, adjust or end the bondage scenario.

---

11 Shay Tiziano and Stefanos Tiziano, "Circulation," *Remedial Ropes* (blog), http://www.remedialropes.com/basic-bondage-safety/circulation/.

**Nerve damage:** Nerve damage is one of the biggest concerns associated with bondage. It can be very tricky to identify because the signs of it tend to vary considerably from person to person. Some people have nerves that absorb and perhaps enjoy a great deal of pain, and others have extremely sensitive ones. The only way to determine this is trial and error (unless the rope bottom happens to know already). Always remember that it is extremely easy to damage nerves. Simple acts such as overextending an arm, tying a rope too tightly so that it crushes or compresses the nerve, or even rubbing against or rolling over a vulnerable nerve with bondage material can cause harm ranging from minor to severe.[12] There are several generally recognized indications of nerve damage. Among these are pain (anywhere from slight to sharp/shooting pain), loss of feeling, electrical sensation (tingling), and loss of nerve signal resulting in weakness (such as loss of grip). Everyone from novices to experienced practitioners should be aware that nerve damage can happen almost instantaneously. If any of these symptoms are experienced, they should be addressed immediately by removing the bondage in order to prevent or minimize damage.

According to rope enthusiast Shay Tiziano,[13] there are six basic factors that contribute to nerve injury:

- **Nerve vulnerability:** Discussed above.
- **Anatomical location (where on the body you are binding):** Joints and the upper arms, for example, are far more risky to tie than the thighs or ankles.
- **Duration of compression:** Removing bondage at the first sign of symptoms may stop the nerve damage from

---

12 Shay Tiziano and Stefanos Tiziano, "Nerve Damage," *Remedial Ropes* (blog), http://www.remedialropes.com/nerve-damage/.

13 Shay Tiziano and Stefanos Tiziano, "Six Contributing Factors to Nerve Damage in Bondage, aka 'The Six Horsepeople of the Nervepocalypse,'" *Remedial Ropes* (blog), http://www.remedialropes.com/bondage-safety-articles/nervepocalypse/.

progressing to more serious stages. The longer you wait, the more damage may occur. Therefore it is important to act on symptoms of nerve damage at the earliest possible opportunity.

- **Severity of compression:** Certain activities, such as suspension bondage and predicament bondage, skew toward increased severity of compression and risk of rope friction, making them inherently more risky.
- **Stretch/stress positioning:** Be mindful that some folks are more flexible and resilient than others and that this can greatly contribute to determining comfort. Some positions are also more likely to lead to nerve damage, either by stretching or stressing the body. Be careful when you try new positions—make sure they are comfortable and safe for your body or the body of your partner.
- **Environment:** Environmental factors that might affect bondage and the ability to release someone quickly include temperature, weather, noise levels, visibility, and the presence or absence of others.

Nerve damage typically lasts anywhere from a few days to three months, and it should be expected to limit if not interrupt use of the injured limb until it heals. In more severe cases of nerve damage, surgery might be required to graft, repair, or replace the nerve if it does not regenerate naturally. Account for the risk factors by negotiating an allowable risk budget and checking in frequently. Empower your partner to communicate with you and address any discomfort rapidly. In case unbinding needs to occur instantaneously, be sure that you always have a reliable, safe cutting implement within reach, and know when and how to safely use it.

**Muscle cramping:** Holding the same position for a long period of time can cause muscles to cramp. Although most muscle cramps are pretty harmless, they are quite painful, so making sure that you're well hydrated and that you've had enough potassium can help to alleviate this. Stretching and warming up the muscles before beginning a bondage scene can also help to prevent cramping during a session. I know (from personal experience) that you might feel compelled to rush through the stretching process to get to the fun stuff, but take my word for it and enjoy a long, luxurious warm-up. Your muscles, and your bondage Top, will thank you for it.

**Light-headedness/fainting:** Light-headedness can happen for a number of reasons: adrenaline rushes, feelings such as anxiety or fear, dehydration or low blood sugar, illness, use of drugs/alcohol, sleep deprivation, low blood pressure, etc. Light-headedness is more likely to happen in standing positions, especially when the hands are raised above the head. It also can occur if the rib cage is constricted with a bondage device and the lungs are unable to expand to their full capacity. The range of experiences scales from dizziness and light-headedness to nausea, vomiting, and fainting, all of which can cause a play partner to fall. Due to risk of falling, *NEVER tie off someone's neck or genitals to a hard point.* Always have backup plans for repositioning nearby, if not built in. For instance, I often tie standing people to a pole so that if they get dizzy they have something to support them as they slide to the ground. I also tend to keep yoga mats or soft rugs on the ground for people to lie on. When working with bottoms who are older or have less mobility, I keep higher chairs or tables nearby to facilitate a smoother level transition, or simply tie in a bed to avoid level transitions altogether.

**Falling:** When I was a child, I learned how to fall safely: "Put your arms out in front of you to brace your fall!" But what do you do when someone falls and their arms are tied behind their back? If someone cannot protect themselves from falling due to their bondage, or if they fall while a limb or body part is still tied off to a hard point, very serious injuries, including death, can occur. At their most innocent, falls can produce bruises or broken bones, and at their worst, they can lead to joint damage, torn ligaments, head injuries, spinal-cord injuries, and death. Falling is one of the biggest risks associated with suspension, so special care should be taken to assure that hard points being used for suspension are safe for load bearing, and that equipment is sound. Someone doesn't have to be in the air to incur risk of falling; standing with the legs or ankles tied or impaired in any way, being off balance, or being perched on a piece of furniture also increase the risk of falling. Another way to minimize the risks of falling is by not tying on hard surfaces, or by padding them with mats, rugs, mattresses, etc.[14]

**Marking:** It is possible for marking or bruising to occur anywhere that a bondage device is used. Know how easily your partner bruises, and to decrease the risk of marking, avoid tightening bondage devices too much or putting too much weight on them.

**Asphyxiation/suffocation:** Lack of oxygen to the brain can cause accidental death. This risk has particularly devastating consequences in terms of mortality and legality. Besides the fact that you could severely brain damage or kill yourself or your partner, legally the act could be considered suicide or murder

---

14 Pete Riggs, "The Safety Series Part 1: Physical Risk with Rope Bondage," *Rope Connections* (blog), July 31, 2015, https://www.ropeconnections.com/the-safety-series-part-1-physical-risk-with-rope-bondage/.

and therefore come with a slew of judicial implications. To avoid asphyxiation, stay away from tying or binding the neck. In the case of a collar, simply leave it loose enough that it does not cause discomfort, and do not tie it off to a hard point, especially if nobody is going to be around to monitor. Gags are not likely to cause asphyxiation, but it is possible that someone could choke on the spit that they produce. Therefore, people who are gagged should always be monitored closely and never left alone. Make sure that bondage that restricts or restrains the chest (such as a harness or corset) is not so tight that it constricts the rib cage and prevents the lungs from expanding. This can also cause someone to pass out. The last potential cause for asphyxiation is a medical emergency such as an asthma or allergy attack without access to an inhaler or EpiPen. This is one of the reasons that discussing medical status is important during negotiation.

**Unforeseen events:** Unfortunately none of us are clairvoyant (if you are, call me—I've got a job for you!). This means that situations and scenarios that we did not plan for can arise during playtime. These types of things include medical emergencies, environmental emergencies, and untimely visitors (the UPS guy really likes delivering to my house because of all the bondage scenes he's accidentally walked in on!). In all seriousness, in any of these scenarios, you'll want to be able to remove bondage as fast as possible. It's important to discuss your risk budget during negotiation and account for whatever you decide. Some tips: Locking someone in a cage overnight in a place that is not easily accessible (without an escape contingency) is a fire or weather emergency hazard. Not only are bondage devices (latex, natural-fiber rope) made from particularly sensitive allergenic materials, but the cleaners and maintenance solutions (beeswax, oils, polishes) used on them could also trigger someone's allergic response. Curtains, locking doors, and sometimes a quickly tossed blanket can do wonders to create a cloak of invisibility around your pervy activities. Make sure to implement a "call before you visit" rule with friends and family if you know that bondage is on the itinerary.

**Predatory behavior:** I was very lucky to begin my bondage exploration in a household of experts who held my safety and well-being in the highest regard. Even when I ventured away from the household for bondage events or parties, my guardians vetted every potential play partner of mine. I'm glad that they did—it saved me from a number of shady situations and potential disasters. I know that my situation was ideal, and that most people don't have access to such a wonderful security system. If you do not have a vetting system, it is advisable that you set up a "safe call" system with a friend to check in. Let them know where you're going, whom you'll be with, and what time to expect a call from you. If they do not hear from you by the agreed-upon time, they should call the authorities. There are many smartphone apps (such as bSafe and Kitestring) that are programmed specifically for personal safety. Install them on your phone.

It is important for you to know that there are people out there who can hurt you whether you are a Top or a bottom. There are novice folks whose excitement or egos convince them that they are more skilled than they really are. There are also folks who have misunderstandings about consent, or simply choose to ignore the topic. Perhaps the most egregious are those who possess both a wealth of knowledge on bondage and a malicious intent—wolves in sheep's clothing. While little can be done to evade a talented sociopath, making sure to engage in a thorough negotiation, as well as a vetting of your potential partner through referrals, can help to intercept predators before they get too close.

### *Personal Accountability*

There are a number of factors such as honesty, intention, and respect, with which you must take personal accountability in regards to safety. Whether you are the Top or the bottom, it is your responsibility to openly and honestly communicate all relevant information to your partner. Do not blame them for not asking! It is especially important that you are honest with yourself and your partners about your experience level, as this can account for differences in the safety procedure.

As far as intention goes, it's important that you make a vow to do no harm to those with whom you engage in bondage activities. There's a difference between imposing dominance or inflicting pain and doing harm. Whether done intentionally or due to miscalculation, causing someone unwanted emotional or physical harm is never going to turn out well. Make sure that you negotiate thoroughly and do your best to adhere to those negotiations. Repeat offenses are considered to be a red flag of a bully or abusive partner and can earn you a bad reputation, or, worse, a criminal record.

Another topic to consider in terms of intention is emotional labor. Do not begin a session with a play partner unless you are prepared to attend to both their physical and emotional needs. BDSM play can lead people into emotionally sensitive as well as altered states of consciousness, so make sure that you're ready to go there with someone before entering into a play scenario with them. Along those lines, take care of and respect your own mental health, too. It is best not to engage in bondage activities when feeling unstable or unfocused.

Finally, respect your partner's wishes in regards to privacy. *Never* out somebody by posting photos of them in bondage devices without their consent, or by any other means. Be considerate of who is in the background when taking photos in a crowded space, and who is within earshot when discussing sensitive matters. Not everyone is able to be out about their alternative lifestyles, and you should be considerate of that.

## TL;DR

Okay, I know that was a lot of information to process, and we are almost done. Here are some quick checklists of do and don't suggestions for aspiring bondage Tops and bottoms. Don't you dare skip the beginning of this chapter and just read this section!

***Bottoms:***

- Only participate in play scenarios with the positive consent of your partner.
- Negotiate your activities and limits with your partner in advance of play.
- Inform your Top about your mental and physical health history before being bound.
- Research the physical risks associated with the type of bondage you are participating in, and check that the appropriate safety tools are immediately accessible during play.
- Don't engage in BDSM activities while under the influence of drugs or alcohol.
- Have a safe-call or contingency plan in place in case things go awry.
- Warm up by stretching before being bound, and move slowly when coming out of bondage.
- Communicate as clearly as possible throughout the bondage experience.
- Know your limitations with regards to pain tolerance, nerve sensitivity, and physical rigor, and voice them assertively.

- Feel empowered to end a play scenario that has crossed a personal limit.

***Tops:***

- Only participate in play scenarios with the positive consent of your partner.
- Negotiate your activities and limits with your partner in advance of play.
- Research the physical risks associated with the type of bondage you are participating in, and ensure that the appropriate safety tools are immediately accessible during play.
- Never leave a bound partner alone and unsupervised.
- Train in bondage techniques before trying advanced techniques (through a class or trusted mentor).
- Never attach rope from the neck or genitals to a hard point.
- Check in frequently with your bottom, and immediately take steps to address potential nerve damage or symptoms of impaired circulation.
- Don't fear that you are checking in too much—your bottom will probably experience check-ins as charming, comforting, or even arousing.
- As you construct a bondage scenario, imagine the consequences if the bottom were to fall. If the answer seems too dangerous, adjust the bondage scenario.
- Avoid large amounts of tension on your partner's joints (such as the armpits, wrists, elbows, knees, or groin).
- Learn how to avoid sensitive nerves.
- Feel empowered to end a play scenario that has crossed a personal limit.

## Communication

As important as negotiation is prior to play, it does not eradicate the necessity of communication during a scene. Communication becomes more important once a bondage scene has begun. Clear and effective communication can account for the time-sensitive differences between injury-free and life-threatening situations. On a less heavy note, clear communication can account for the difference between knowing just how to push someone's buttons and feeling lost about how to make them feel good. Why grasp at straws or suffer in silence rather than tell your partner what's up? Even if you do want to communicate, you might feel tongue-tied due to a lack of experience in talking about this aspect of your sexuality. As your guide, I would like to offer you some tips for both verbal and nonverbal communication during bondage scenes. Both are important, especially because bondage can involve gags that prevent speech and/or venues with loud volumes that stifle verbal communication. It is important that no matter what your environment or what the scenario you're involved in, you are able to communicate clearly and effectively.

### *Verbal Communication*

You should feel comfortable communicating clearly with your partner about any discomfort, needs, or desires that you have during play ("Can you shift that cuff downward a little more, please?" "My hands are beginning to tingle." "I'm going to let you out soon." "Would you please tease my cunt while I'm tied like this?" etc.). Feelings matter, so communicating clearly and effectively also means considerately. Try not to put your partner down or sound accusatory when communicating with them ("You always tie that too tight" versus "Would you mind tying that more loosely from now on?"). In certain scenarios, it's important to expedite the communication process, especially when safety is on the line. In these types of situations, verbal communication systems such as safewords, pain scales, and number and color systems can be used to speed things up without sacrificing clarity. Using communication systems might take some getting used to, but with practice has the potential to facilitate clear and effective communication with ease.

**Safewords:** A safeword is a signal word that a bottom can use to communicate their physical or emotional needs to a Top. I like to think of safewords as safety mechanisms, like the airbags in your car—even if you don't use them, it makes you feel better to know that they're there. Generally, safewords are used when approaching, reaching, or crossing a boundary or limit. Just because you discussed what the boundaries were during negotiation does not mean that your partner will be able to magically identify when you're reaching that boundary. As previously stated, as partners get to know each other more, they might have less need for safewords, but it never hurts to have a contingency plan when it comes to the well-being of a loved one. To avoid using safewords accidentally, assigned safewords should be words that wouldn't typically arise during a sexual or bondage scenario. That doesn't mean they have to be nonsense words, and in fact, I think they shouldn't be. Because safewords are meant to be used as safety mechanisms in a moment of stress, shouting out "banana" or "pumpernickel" might cause the Top to laugh, when what is needed in that moment is focus and sensitivity. My favorite safeword is actually the phrase "Please show mercy" (or just "mercy" for short, although you'd be surprised how fast those three words can fly out of someone's mouth!). Because I am attracted to D/s dynamics, that is the easiest way for me or my bottom to indicate that we're experiencing difficulty while maintaining the protocol of the relationship. "Safetunes" can be used in instances where a gag might interrupt the bottom's ability to enunciate. Even with a gag in the mouth, it is possible to hum a specific tune that indicates that your bottom needs help. For the purposes of expediency, only have them sing a few notes rather than a ballad. Typically though, it's best to use a hierarchical safeword system, especially with unfamiliar partners. The most popular safeword system in the BDSM scene is the stoplight system, wherein "green" means go, "yellow" indicates that you're approaching a boundary, and "red" initiates a hard stop to all activities.

**Pain scale:** The pain scale is a tool that is generally used in medical scenarios to measure a patient's pain. Your partner can be asked to ascribe a number to their experience, ranging from zero ("no hurt") to ten ("hurts worst"). This type of communication system can be useful when using new implements or engaging with new partners, as everyone processes pain differently, and it can be difficult, even for the most experienced players, to assess what their partner is feeling without feedback.

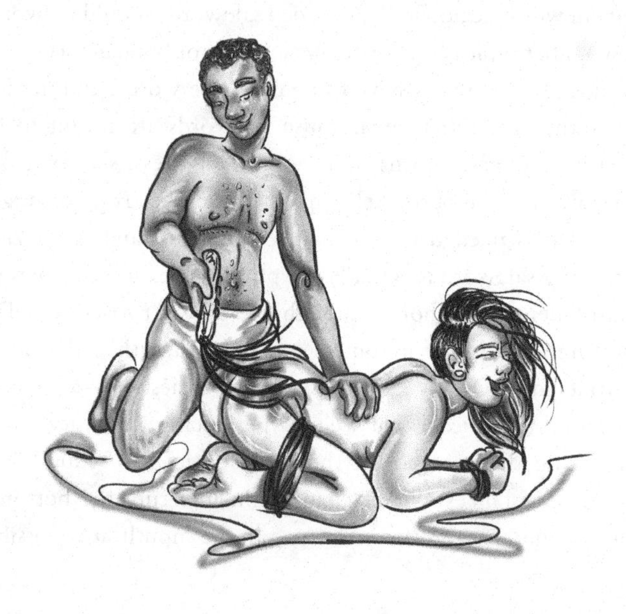

**Number/color system:** The number/color system was created by a play partner of mine, Andi Buch, by combining the concept of the stoplight safeword system and the pain scale. Some might find this extensive of a system to be overkill, but as I mentioned earlier, it can be very beneficial to overcommunicate when wading into the territory of bondage play, and this is a great tool for that.

What Andi's system does is extend the stoplight safeword system mentioned above into a more full spectrum, wherein color equates to a fully realized spectrum of intolerance and pleasure. The system is intuitive in many ways. It extends the already universally known stoplight-safeword system. It does so in an intuitive manner by using a very well-known color wheel or rainbow. The best part about it is that communications in this system need only a single word to be effective. As such, it is extremely efficient and easy to use, regardless of how incoherent a bottom's headspace may be. Moreover, as a Top, you can ask, "Color?" and immediately have reference for where your bottom's headspace is.

> RED: Stop. No more. I need what is happening to stop.
> ORANGE: I'm about to call red. I really can't take any more of this. Change what you're doing, please.
> YELLOW: Meh . . . this isn't really working for me, but I can tolerate it.
> GREEN: Okay, everything's fine. Thanks for checking in :)
> BLUE: Oooh, this is fun! Yes, please, more of this!
> PURPLE: Oh my goddess this is amazing!
> ULTRAVIOLET: THISISTHEBESTTHINGIVEEVERFELTHOLYF★CKKK

While this color system is useful, it's limited to one axis, that of intolerance and enjoyment. Thus, the model suggests adding a second axis to the equation: that of numbers (one to ten) to indicate level of intensity.

So, for instance, in a flogging scene, these numbers might map something like:

1: I can barely feel the flogger at all
5: This is starting to get a bit painful
10: My skin feels like it's on fire.

Note that this is an altogether different spectrum from what the colors are being used to reference. For instance, while most of us would equate a ten with red, an intense, hard-core masochist might find a ten to be ultraviolet for them.

On the flip side, while most of us wouldn't mind a one, a person with fibromyalgia might find incredibly light touches intolerably red.

These two axes give us a simple vocabulary with which to relay a number of different states as a bottom, and to efficiently inquire ("Color and number, please?") as a Top. Having it at your fingertips will do wonders to open your comfortability as a Top, and to help you effectively communicate in any scene.

### *Nonverbal Communication*

In addition to verbal communication systems, nonverbal communication systems are important to have in place for a variety of reasons including accessibility, reliability, and ease of communication.

**Reading body language:** While reading body language is intuitive for some, it can be helpful to learn a few telltale physical indicators of your partner's emotional state. Things like muscle tension, stiffness, raised shoulders, curling of the spine, and grimacing should tell you that your partner is struggling, whereas hip grinding and heavy breathing indicate that they're aroused. Reading body language should not be considered to be universal, as gesticulation varies from one person to the next. Paying close attention to your partner's body language while using verbal communication systems will help you to learn their movements and how their body reacts to different stimuli. With practice, you'll be able to recognize your partner's state by the movements of their body rather than having to listen for a number, color, or other vocal cue. While this is not a foolproof system, it does provide for deeply empathetic connections between partners, and for that reason it is one of my favorite modes of communication.

**Hand squeezing:** Hand squeezing is a useful communication system for bondage scenarios because it doesn't require mobility or even use of the mouth to communicate. Most types of bondage (except for mummification and encasement) should allow for one hand to be accessible to the Top. Squeezing is used to check for nerve safety, because if the radial nerve is compressed too much either around the upper arm or at the wrist, the ability to close the hand will become impaired. Squeezing your partner's hand before they are bound will tell you what their normal grip feels like. Place your fingers inside their hand once they are bound and let them squeeze again. As long as they can produce a similar grip, at least their radial nerves are not being compressed too much. If the pressure in their grip changes, adjust the bondage immediately. You can also use a series of secret handshakes, squeezes, or Morse code–like pulses of the fingers to indicate status or safewords. I use one quick squeeze for red and two hard squeezes for green. Others have been known to use squeezes to indicate where they are on the pain scale, or they've even set up more elaborate handshake/hand signal systems.

**Token object:** Token objects can be held in the hand, mouth, or anywhere else that the bottom has control over. These should be bright objects that are easily visible, as they are meant to flag the Top and indicate a safeword. Usually, I like to use handkerchiefs, bells, feathers, or even a paddle that I've been using during the scene. I let the bottom hold on to it and tell them to let go if they need to get my attention. If I see the object fall to the floor, I immediately stop what I'm doing and check in with them. This can be a very helpful system to use in a crowded dungeon or loud venue.

## Aftercare

BDSM play can be incredibly intense, so after sharing a bondage experience with your partner, it's important to take some time to tend to both of your emotional and physical needs. First, tend to any first aid that is necessary and make sure that both the Top and bottom are hydrated. Then you can move on to more in-depth aftercare. For some people that means cuddling and holding their partner close, while others desire alone time or space to process. What ideal aftercare looks like for you should be discussed during negotiation. If you're someone who requires alone time to process but your partner desires physical closeness, it might be appropriate to assign a surrogate cuddler such as a pet, stuffed animal, or trusted friend. This is especially important when someone has bottomed and feels that they want or need physical closeness to help process a scene. Other wonderful forms of aftercare involve taking a bath or shower together, giving massages, eating your favorite foods, journaling, or simply having a conversation about what you just experienced together. Engaging immediate aftercare is not always possible, but it does make a huge difference in the experience. I recommend that you budget some time for it as often as you are able to. If time constraints prevent you from doing this, it is still advisable to check in with your bondage partner in person or by telephone or virtual means in the days following your experience together. Being present for and attentive to someone's needs is a part of the process of being bound to or bound by them.

## Why do people engage in bondage activities?

Hopefully by now you've had time to process the complex terminology and important concepts that were covered in the previous sections, and your curiosity is piqued. After the module on safety protocols, you might find yourself thinking that if there's so much risk involved with erotic bondage activities, why on earth do people choose to engage in them? I'm here to tell you that the answers to that question are vast. I probably can't provide every single answer to that question within the pages of this book, but what I will attempt to do is hold a candle to some of the bondage experiences that we all share. Many of them are hiding in plain sight! Because you likely haven't thought of these seemingly innocent topics as forms of bondage before, some of them might seem shocking or even upsetting to you. That's okay. I often urge people to pay just as much attention to the things that attract them as those that repel them. Often, your reactions tell you far more about yourself than the subject matter at hand. So, with that piece of advice, keep an open mind, and please continue reading.

### *The Shared Wombic Experience*

No matter who we are or where we come from, we all share the same first bondage experience—being bound within the safe confines of the womb, literally tethered to our mothers via the umbilical cord. While it might not be very sexy to think about bondage in this context, doing so explains a lot about why people enjoy the sensations of restraint and encasement.

Floating in the cushion of amniotic fluid inside the uterus, we are all informed by our senses. As early as eleven weeks into pregnancy, we, as fetuses, develop the sensation of touch, and we begin to explore the boundaries of our own bodies and the womb that encapsulates us. Ultrasound scans taken during this time show babies "touching their buttocks, holding onto the umbilical cord, turning and walking up and down the amniotic sac wall on the inside,"[15] according to Heidelise Als, associate professor of psychology at Harvard Medical School and Children's Hospital Boston. We are not still and quiet in the womb as many believe; on the contrary, we exist to explore the variety of sensations that life has to offer.

Als believes that fetuses use touch to both soothe and teach themselves.

"Fetuses are laying down their own cortical networks in the brain. . . . When babies are born prematurely . . . you will see these little preemies trying to bring their hands together or bring their hands to their face, or lay them over their head and their ear. . . . They search, literally, with their feet to try to find a boundary."[16]

What we learn from these poor little preemie babies (I was one of them!) is that knowing where our boundaries are is soothing to us. The cute feeling that expecting mothers often describe as the baby kicking might actually be the baby trying to locate and hold boundaries. An overly firm touch on a pregnant belly is known to cause the baby to move away or stick out their arm as if to hold a boundary. Likewise, a delicate or gentle touch creates a reaction that seems to welcome the sensation across the boundary. From the moment that we learn to feel, boundaries become incredibly important to us. We identify the boundaries

---

15 Camilla Cornell, "Fetal development: What your baby's up to in the womb," *Today's Parent*, March 14, 2011, https://www.todaysparent.com/pregnancy/being-pregnant/what-does-my-baby-do-in-the-womb/.

16 Ibid.

of our own skin and the lush space that envelops us. This is the beginning of our adventure with bondage.

Other senses such as taste and hearing are developed and honed within the womb. These senses contribute to emotional bonding with the outside world, by allowing us to hear the voices of our parents, taste the foods our mother is eating, and grow accustomed to sensations that we will experience once we've entered the world. We will look for the familiar to soothe us once we've left the womb. The environment inside the womb is so perfect for an unborn child that it influences our preferences for the rest of our lives.

When our mother's water breaks, the membrane that holds the amniotic fluid that we were floating in ruptures. This signal that the baby is coming is also the destruction of the world as we knew it. Our first boundary disappears in a flash, and we are squeezed through a tight canal, out into the open world. Our reward for entering this brand-new terrain? The umbilical cord that carried oxygen and nutrients to us inside the womb, the literal tie to our mothers, is cut. In doing so, we break free from the boundaries of our mother's body and create a new physical boundary of our own. What an exciting day!

To aid with the overwhelming sensation of being in a completely new environment, and the loss of connection to our mothers, we are swaddled in blankets or clothes. This helps to mimic the sensation of being inside the womb, keeping us calm and warm. Most babies love to be swaddled, but the ones that don't still enjoy being held tightly by their parents. Being held by our parents, touched, fed, and cared for constitute emotional bonding. Even though the physical bonds no longer exist between us and our mothers, feeling their skin against ours is incredibly soothing for us both and allows for us to grow closer together.[17]

---

17 Larissa Hirsch, MD, "Bonding With Your Baby," *KidsHealth* (blog), June 2015, https://kidshealth.org/en/parents/bonding.html.

When you think about it in this context, you can see why simply even coming into existence is related to bondage. We break free from our physical bonds to become our own people, and once we do, we seek the comfort and safety that we experienced within the womb. Emotional bonds with loved ones help to provide that for us until we are old enough to start seeking out those sources of comfort on our own. No wonder so many of us enjoy practicing restraint with our lovers! Whether we are conscious of it or not, it reminds us of our wombic experience and provides the comfort that we've sought since coming into the world.

#### *Recreating the wombic experience through restraint*

Just as mothers create life by delivering children from the confines of their bodies into the open air, we can give birth to new ideas, experiences, and levels of understanding through our exploration of bondage. The theme of drawing thoughts and feelings that are buried deep inside us out into the light where we can see them is a recurring one in the exploration of bondage. As adults, we don't often have the opportunities to express our innermost feelings and desires. In many cases, we become unaware of them because we live in an age when business and distraction are lauded and held above self-exploration. People are constantly on the go, buzzing from one activity to the next, rarely stopping to smell the flowers. However, when the body is restrained or controlled through discipline, the mind becomes free to explore.

Similar to the confines of the womb, restraint though bondage devices forces us to determine the boundaries of our bodies. It's a particularly useful mindfulness tool in erotic contexts because it affects our sense of proprioception, or the awareness of where all of our body parts are in relation to one another, and to the world. This is our first step toward recreating the wombic experience.

Proprioception is the reason you know where your right pinkie toe is right now even though you aren't looking at it or touching it. It is also the reason that you can walk, tie your shoes, type, or drive a car. In fact, proprioception contributes to committing actions to muscle memory, thus making tasks that once required concentration feel like they've been "programmed" into your body over time. Erotic play, like these other activities, requires the use of the body in ways that can take some getting used to. Traditional intercourse, for example, might feel uncomfortable at first but with repetition becomes an activity that can be enjoyed without worrying about the mechanics. However, unlike tying your shoes, actions becoming second nature during erotic play can set someone back. This is because erotic play is usually more enjoyable if you're aware of what your body is feeling, and that is where restraint comes into play.

Restraint can highlight the limitations of the body by restricting movement of body parts that are usually able to move freely, or simply by providing sensory awareness to where the boundaries of the body are in space. When you are bound, you are held. Skin is no longer the outermost layer that contains you. The sensation of rope, leather, or other bondage tools on the skin informs you about the new rules and restrictions that have been set. They control your reality and act as an extension of the dominant partner who has dreamed up your new landscape. Sound familiar? Practicing restraint allows us to revisit the process of creation in an erotic context, and unlike when we are in the womb, it allows us to be in control of our own experience.

Sensory awareness can also be explored through restraint. The sensation of pressure that is produced by bondage invokes the sensations we experienced by floating in the amniotic fluid, being squeezed through the birth canal, and being swaddled and rocked by our caretakers. The sensation of pressure on our skin or bodies is known to trigger the release of the mood-enhancing neurotransmitters serotonin and dopamine.[18] In other words, it soothes us and makes us feel good. The "restraint" or deprivation of other senses such as sight or hearing can also provide pleasurable results. When one sense is dampened, the mind relies more heavily upon the others, making the input from those senses more noticeable than usual. As such, restraint affects the physical body in two ways; it introduces new sensations and heightens others. In a process similar to the sensory learning that occurs within the womb, one's physical experience informs the mental one. Paying attention to these new and unusual sensations and how they affect our psychological/emotional landscapes can be incredibly rich and fulfilling opportunities for discovery.

### *Social motivators for experiencing bondage*

Don't panic—our shared experience in the womb does not account for all of the reasons that we enjoy bondage activities. Once we are brought into the world and begin to explore it, we find many other examples of bondage in plain sight!

Society, in and of itself, produces a unique form of bondage for us to grapple with. We come from a history of thousands of years of nonconsensual power exchange dynamics that are imposed upon us by social structure. No matter where you come from on the planet, if you trace back far enough in history, you will find examples of kings and serfs, pharaohs and slaves, haves and have-nots. Though we do not choose to be born into these roles, we are expected to adhere to them. Especially in today's unpredictable political climate, adhering to the social roles assigned to us can be incredibly painful, frustrating, and downright dangerous. By engaging in consensual power exchange with loved ones, we can let go of socially deemed roles by stepping into a different

---

18 Alescia Ford-Lanza, MS OTR/L, ATP, "The Ultimate Guide to Deep Pressure Therapy," *Special Needs* (blog), *Harkla*, May 25, 2017, https://harkla.co/blogs/special-needs/deep-pressure-therapy.

role than the one chosen for us. Even if just for a few hours in the bedroom, the most socially powerless person can experience the feeling of being in charge, and the most socially powerful person can experience subjugation and ego deflation. We can also use consensual power exchange to embrace the parts of our socially deemed roles that we enjoy without having to feel guilty about it (i.e., "But I'm a feminist; why do I enjoy feeling subjugated?"). In doing so, engaging in consensual erotic bondage becomes a form of sociopolitical resistance.

Engaging in consensual erotic bondage can also be connected to religion for some practitioners. The word "religion" actually comes from a Latin word meaning "to bind fast."[19] The idea behind the term *religion* is that the devotee is bound under an obligation to the god/goddess of their choosing. Just by looking at Abrahamic religions, you'll see that both the Old and New Testaments are rife with bondage references (both consensual and nonconsensual). I have known many people whose early exposures to the concept of bondage involved looking at a crucifix on the wall. Mine might have been learning about the Jews being delivered from bondage at the Passover seder. Many people repurpose familiar religious concepts (such as prayer, fasting, and chastity) and items (such as crucifixes, holy water, and tefillin) in erotic bondage as aids to sexual exploration in order to express spiritual agency, defiance, or even rebellion.

Other forms of social bondage include the beauty standards or gender roles imposed on us. Just think about how many children are ascribed a gender (along with color preferences for clothing and acceptable toys for them to play with) before they are able to express their personal affinities. Gender comes with a whole set of rules about what we're allowed to wear and not wear, do and not do. Some bondage devices such as corsets and

---

19 *Online Etymology Dictionary*, s.v. "Religion," accessed November 25, 2017, https://www.etymonline.com/word/religion.

high-heeled shoes were created for the purpose of adhering to these social mores, bending and shaping the body as society deemed aesthetically fit. In today's culture of gender exploration, gender nonconformists have adopted these bondage devices and techniques to shape their own bodies in the ways that they prefer. People with breasts who desire a more masculine appearance have been known to bind their breasts to their chest. People who desire a shapelier hourglass figure use corsetry and high-heeled shoes, whether or not society deems that as appropriate. Shapeshifting by repurposing items that were once meant to oppress human expression is another way of breaking free from the chains of socially enforced bondage.

Simply existing in the world predicates experiencing trauma. Life is not a picnic, and no matter who we are, we experience unpleasant and sometimes devastating events. Whether your trauma begins with a lowercase or capital *T* might determine how much you want to explore it on your own or with the help of a therapist. Either way, revisiting sensations that were experienced during a traumatic event in a consent-oriented manner can allow for the reclamation of bodily autonomy. Keep in mind that revisiting traumatic events is often triggering in very intense ways. Engaging with our shadow side is never easy, and if you're looking for a therapeutic experience, you should really do so with the help of a trained professional.

Outside of processing trauma, there are myriad psychological motivations for engaging in consensual bondage activities, the biggest one being the emotional bonding that it encourages. Being restrained, albeit consensually, imposes a great sense of vulnerability onto our bodies. Vulnerability here does not mean the act of being weak—on the contrary, it implies the courage to be yourself, and to allow yourself to be fully seen by your partner(s). Being vulnerable involves uncertainty, risk, and emotional exposure, and therefore requires a great deal of trust.

However, to know that you are seen and loved for who you are, and to witness someone else in all of their vulnerability and love them for it, might just be one of life's most fulfilling experiences. It is through engaging in bondage that we are able to replicate the unconditional love we once received from our parents with partners of our own choosing.

Bondage activities can also be incredibly meditative. Because we are accustomed to being able to move about or scratch our own itches, immobility concentrates the mind in a unique manner. While many people find it to be frustrating at first, by breathing and relaxing into restraint, we can literally alter our brain waves, and therefore our consciousness. Through bondage, we can explore aspects of ourselves that we never knew existed.

### Physical motivators for engaging in bondage

Other motivators for engaging in erotic bondage activities include the desire to experience pain or other physical sensations, and to be controlled, subjugated, or erotically stimulated. In other words, they are physical motivations. Bondage devices can be used to caress the body, and erogenous zones in particular, covering the whole spectrum of sensation from pleasure to pain. The placement of knots can cause direct stimulation of the clitoris, perineum, anus, or other areas through simple pressure or through movement across the skin. They can also increase sensitivity by pulling the skin tight and restricting blood flow.

Bondage can also compensate for physical imbalances in a relationship by imposing new physical rules. A stronger partner can be rendered helpless, or a weaker partner can be empowered, inviting an entirely new power dynamic into the relationship. For couples that are accustomed to traditional intercourse, this shift of equality in the bedroom can be quite potent!

### *Recreational motivators for engaging in bondage*

Bondage is a key tool in the activity of erotic role play. Using appropriate restraints can be important in creating the most realistic fantasy for you and your partner to enjoy. As children, we are encouraged to use our imaginations to step outside ourselves and into fantasy, but somewhere along the route to adulthood, role play becomes relegated to the bedroom. Play is important for adults, as it helps us to leave the stressors of our adult lives behind. Without some form of restraint, many games such as prisoner or kidnap scenarios would be missing a major element, so break out the restraints and let those imaginations go wild!

Finally, many forms of bondage, especially Japanese rope bondage, can be considered an art form. Techniques can be honed to adorn and accentuate the beauty of the human body. Plenty of people choose to learn both decorative and restrictive bondage as a recreational or leisure activity that they can share with loved ones. Just like any other art form, learning to control the mediums of bondage in a masterful way takes years, and might turn into a lifelong endeavor.

## What type of bondage is right for you?

As you can see, there are millions of reasons why we as humans might enjoy or choose to engage in bondage. Different types of bondage produce different results, so it is important to consider what goals you're trying to achieve or what outcomes you desire from your bondage experience before choosing a type of bondage activity. The following flow chart has been constructed to help you figure out which type of bondage to engage in based on your mood and personal goals. It can be used as a helpful part of your negotiation process, and then implemented by flipping to that chapter in the book and trying out the tutorials associated with that realm of bondage.

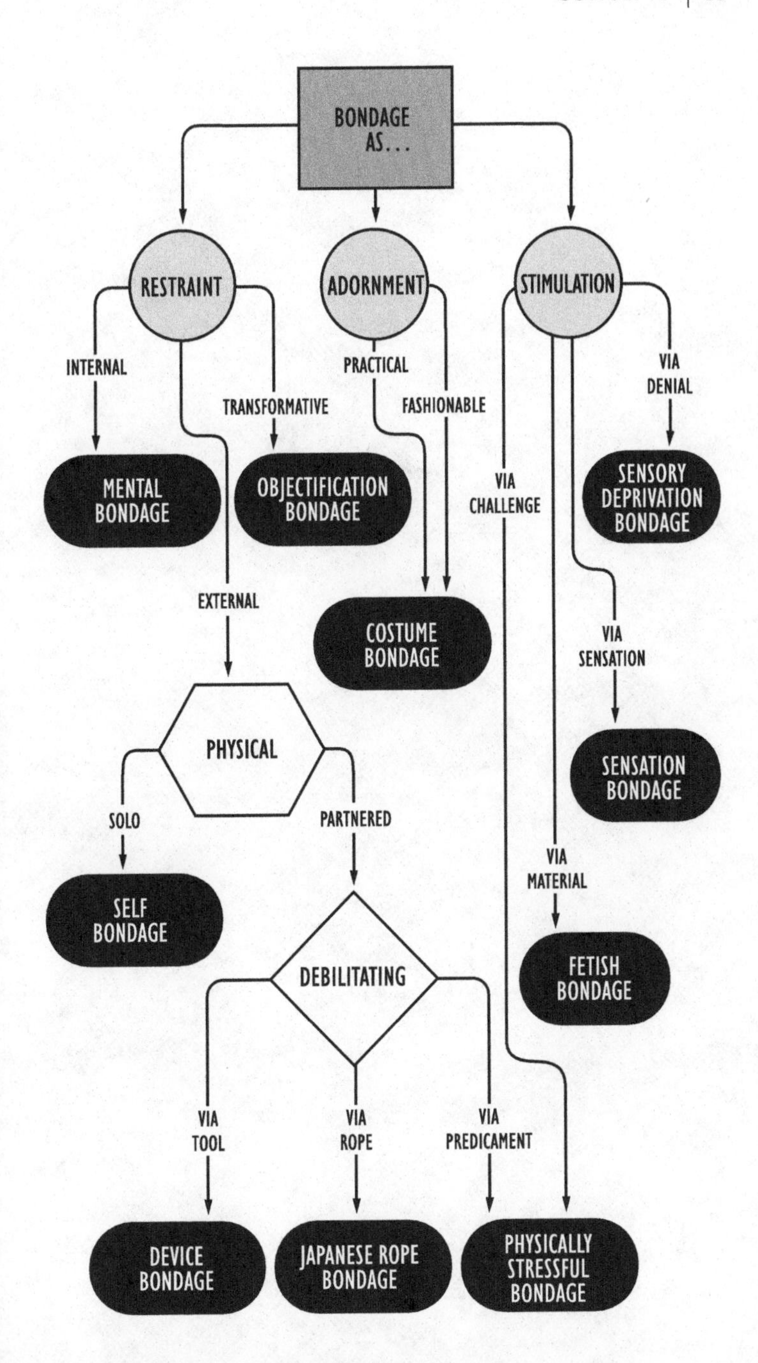
BONDAGE AS...
RESTRAINT
ADORNMENT
STIMULATION
INTERNAL
TRANSFORMATIVE
PRACTICAL
FASHIONABLE
VIA CHALLENGE
VIA DENIAL
MENTAL BONDAGE
OBJECTIFICATION BONDAGE
SENSORY DEPRIVATION BONDAGE
EXTERNAL
COSTUME BONDAGE
VIA SENSATION
PHYSICAL
SENSATION BONDAGE
SOLO
PARTNERED
VIA MATERIAL
SELF BONDAGE
DEBILITATING
FETISH BONDAGE
VIA TOOL
VIA ROPE
VIA PREDICAMENT
DEVICE BONDAGE
JAPANESE ROPE BONDAGE
PHYSICALLY STRESSFUL BONDAGE

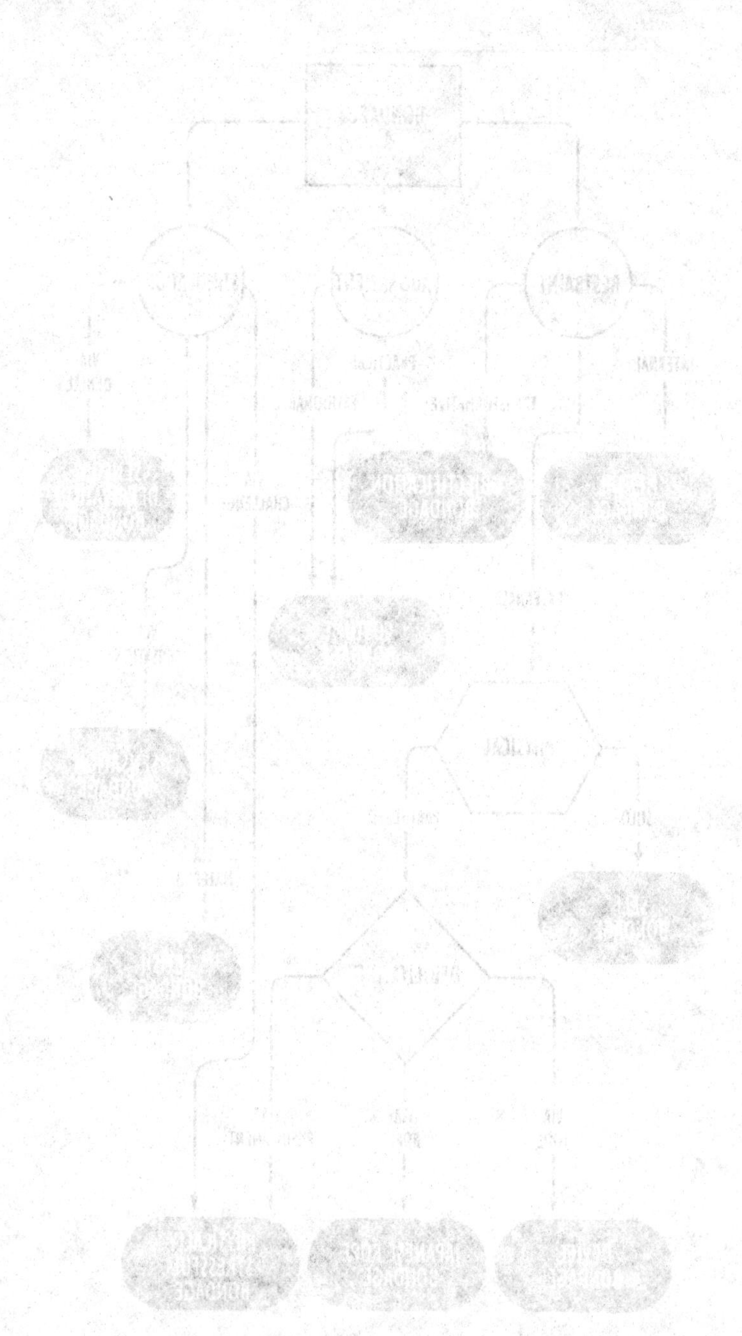

# SECTION 2:

# TEN REALMS OF BONDAGE

In this section, you will read ten chapters about the following types of bondage, originally inspired by Patrick Califia's essay "Bound by Love"[20] and expanded upon based on my own research and thought.

**Japanese rope bondage:** A popular form of rope bondage (which many purport to be the "original" rope bondage technique) that derives from Japanese culture and tradition.

**Device bondage:** Bondage that focuses on the use of tools and devices to enforce restraint. Typically, device bondage is designed to be useful or practical rather than decorative.

**Mental bondage:** A form of bondage that involves mutual agreements or elements of mind control rather than physically imposed restraint.

**Objectification bondage:** Methods of bondage that are implemented with the intention of transforming the bottom into an object or thing. Certain acts of objectification are intended to be degrading and dehumanizing, whereas others aim to build confidence by transforming the subject into an object of desire or commodity.

**Costume bondage:** Methods of bondage that are built into fashion items or clothing so as to appeal to the aesthetic preference of the viewer and heighten the wearer's sense of self-expression. On the surface, costume bondage appears to be used for adornment. However, these clothing items may include additional bondage functions such as constriction, shape-shifting, movement restriction, objectification, and encasement.

---

20 Patrick Califia, "Bound by Love," in *Bondage: An Anthology of Passionate Restraint*, ed. John Warren (Masquerade Books, 1998), 27-48.

**Sensation bondage:** The purpose of sensation bondage is to heighten the bottom's awareness of their own skin and to play with the variety of sensations that bondage tools have to offer.

**Fetish bondage:** Bondage activities wherein participants are able to engage with specific materials that, in and of themselves, arouse the participants.

**Sensory deprivation:** Sensory deprivation is a type of bondage that focuses on restricting one or more of the senses in a way that increases the Top's power over the bottom.

**Physically stressful bondage:** The purpose of physically stressful bondage is to present a challenge in the form of discomfort or pain. It is different from pain bondage in that it forces the bottom to participate in their own torture.

**Self-bondage:** Self-bondage is the use of restraints on oneself for erotic pleasure. Self-bondage can be more risky than partner bondage due to the lack of a spotter.

Each chapter will contain historical, cultural, and practical information about each topic, as well as tutorials for you to try at home. I hope that your exploration continues to be insightful, inspiring, and erotic. Happy reading!

CHAPTER

# 3

# JAPANESE ROPE BONDAGE

The first medium that comes to mind when people hear the word *bondage* is rope. Within the bondage community, rope is considered a bondage essential due to its affordability and versatility. It can be used for restrictive bondage that holds people tightly, decorative bondage that adorns them, and even suspension bondage that dangles them from the ceiling! It is because of this versatility that the bondage community and the images associated with it are dominated by rope. Outside the BDSM community, the *Fifty Shades of Grey* series has greatly contributed to rope bondage becoming normalized as a sexual activity within the eyes of the public. Whereas rope bondage was once widely viewed as subversive or taboo, it is now seen as a novelty. This new attitude toward rope bondage is just another evolution in the extensive history of the practice. As your guide, I would be remiss to jump into information about rope bondage without paying some homage to its traditional Japanese roots.

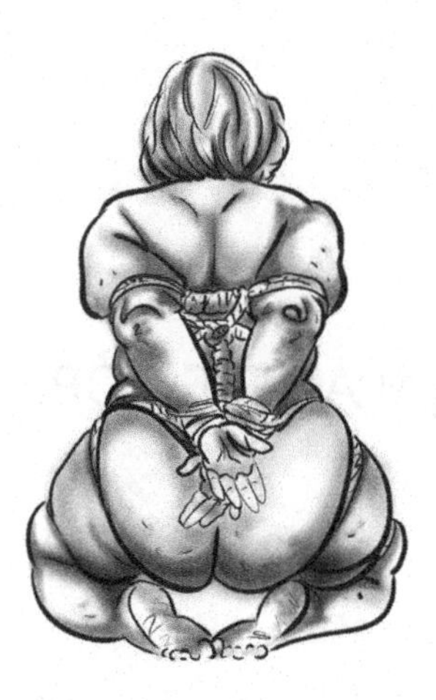

## History of Japanese Rope Bondage

Rope tying and restraint have had countless practical and decorative functions throughout Japan's history. In her book *The Seductive Art of Japanese Bondage*, famed bondage practitioner Midori makes the claim that "the relationship of the Japanese, rope and tying objects . . . [is] possibly as old as the Japanese civilization itself."[21] The evidence of rope in Japanese culture can be traced back to the Jomon period (10,000 BCE to 300 BCE). The term *Jomon* actually means "rope pattern," and receives its name from the rope-patterned pottery that the period is known for. Since that time, rope has been an integral tool in Japanese religious ceremonies, art, clothing, and especially law-enforcement practices.

During a period of brutal warfare known as the Warring States period (approximately 1467–1600), rope-tying techniques became integral in Japanese battle, both as a martial art and a tool of incarceration. The techniques known as *Tasuki-dori* and

21 Midori, *The Seductive Art of Japanese Bondage* (Greenery Press, 2001), loc. 188 of 1168, Kindle.

*Hobako-jutsu* were used for the capture and takedown of an opponent on the move. *Hojo-jutsu* was a more static technique, used to bind a prisoner for the purposes of interrogation or torture. Many of the modern-day bondage patterns and styles that you see in magazines and on the internet are based off the techniques listed above.[22]

The era that followed was the Edo period (1600–1868). It was in this period that newfound peacekeeping procedures and prosperity led to a split in the application of rope arts. One branch of practitioners maintained the practices of the previous era, polishing the martial art techniques, and the other developed artistic and erotic applications of said practices. The first branch became codified in 1742, when the Tokugawa government instituted a legal framework that distinguished seven kinds of punishment. The most extreme punishments were death, exile, slavery, and forced labor. They also instituted rules of torture, with two types of torture that concerned bondage: bending by rope (*ebireme*), and suspension (*isur zeme*).[23] You will read more about why these techniques were so physically challenging in Chapter 11.

The job of capturing criminals was assigned to officials who ranked below the samurai. It's possible the samurai believed that the application of restraint was below their class, since it limited their opponents by handicapping them. The officials who did capture criminals, the doshin, used bondage to convey the nature of the crime, time of capture, and, most importantly, the social status of the prisoners.[24] The doshin used different tying

---

22 Ibid, loc. 202 of 1168.

23 Masami Akita, "Punishment and the Beauty of Japanese Bondage (Kinbaku): The History of S&M in Japan," *Secret Magazine*, April 1997, 53, www.secretmag.com/PDF/Best12.PDF.

24 Masami Akita, "Punishment and the Beauty of Japanese Bondage (Kinbaku): The History of S&M in Japan," *Secret Magazine*, April 1997, 54, www.secretmag.com/PDF/Best12.PDF.

methods and rope colors to create these distinctions.[25] Because of the importance placed on social status, incorrect binding would lead to embarrassment and disgrace to the officials involved. Therefore, methods of binding were strictly upheld by the doshin and generally handed down by oral tradition to those who proved themselves worthy of the privilege. Those who did so were taught tying patterns that were well guarded by their superior mentors.[26] Once the prisoner was bound, another aspect of punishment came into play—public disgrace.

Throughout history, societies have used public disgrace to deter criminal behavior. Such public displays frequently turned into a form of mass entertainment. This was the case by the reign of the fourth and fifth Tokugawa military dictators, during which time criminals were often tied to a horse and paraded through the city. As is frequently the case, the experience of public disgracing was much harder on women. Masajiro commented that male onlookers were aroused by the demeaning display of these female criminals. In Japan, this led inevitably to bondage art that was dominated by images of women tortured by *ebireme* and *isur zeme*.[27] It is no surprise then that the other branch of rope bondage, which centered around the artistic and erotic, was developed using these themes of restraint and subjugation for entertainment purposes.

This other branch of rope art was influenced by the increasing demand for entertainment outside of judicial punishment among the newly affluent middle class. Popularized by Kabuki theater, rope was used to enhance both *nureba* (romance and sex

---

25 Midori, *The Seductive Art of Japanese Bondage* (Greenery Press, 2001), loc. 213 of 1168, Kindle.

26 Masami Akita, "Japanese Bondage Origins 1," Bondage Project. Accessed Dec 1, 2017. http://www.bondageproject.com/public/history_e1.htm.

27 Masami Akita, "Punishment and the Beauty of Japanese Bondage (Kinbaku): The History of S&M in Japan," *Secret Magazine*, April 1997, 53, www.secretmag.com/PDF/Best12.PDF.

scenes) and *semega* (torture scenes).[28] Similar to the trends of the Shakespearean theater in England, these titillating scenes were extremely popular, so with advances in the art of woodblock printing, the images from these scenes started to be proliferated.

Ito Seiu, generally considered one of the fathers of contemporary rope bondage, was a traditional Japanese artist and *semega* master with a style whose foundation is built on the Edo woodblock tradition. Born in 1882 and deceased in 1961, Ito Seiu acted as the perfect bridge between cultural tradition and modern innovation. His artistic eye and personal interest in SM, inspired by childhood fairy tales, led him to begin studying bondage in 1908.[29] Most likely, he trained with others who had learned the art through oral traditions of the Edo period and from there evolved his own style. In 1919, he took his first photographs of "punished women," and by the mid-1920s, Ito's photography could be found in underground S&M photo magazines.[30] The proliferation of these images inspired other artists to follow suit, despite the classification of such materials as smut. Today's highly popularized bondage imagery still contains traces of Ito's original style (especially the trademark tousled hair), but in an interview for *Amatoria* magazine in 1953, he said, "The only recognition I ever received as a person who has studied bondage since 1908, was the pervert tag."[31] Perhaps this was true while he was alive, but in today's bondage circles, Ito Seiu is a name that is revered.

After World War II, Americans brought images of rope bondage back to the United States and popularized them in bondage

---

28 Midori, *The Seductive Art of Japanese Bondage* (Greenery Press, 2001), loc. 223 of 1168, Kindle.

29 Ibid, loc. 230 of 1168.

30 Ibid.

31 Masami Akita, "Punishment and the Beauty of Japanese Bondage (Kinbaku): The History of S&M in Japan," *Secret Magazine*, April 1997, 54, www.secretmag.com/PDF/Best12.PDF.

photo clubs, like Irving Klaw's mail-order cheesecake photos of Bettie Page and John Willie's *Bizarre* magazine. This trend was mirrored in Japan by *Kitan Club*, a pulp magazine edited by Kita Reiko, who claimed to be the "last disciple of bondage master Ito Seiu."[32] As these types of images became more popular across the globe, they enticed a new generation of people to become invested in the art form. Since then, rope bondage has evolved and branched off into even more schools of theory, practice, and application, simultaneously becoming clarified as well as muddled and confused by the general public.

Today, there are two words that are most commonly used to refer to Japanese rope bondage: shibari and kinbaku. *Shibari* means "to tie" in Japanese.[33] The word existed in the Japanese language in a nonwritten form before the Chinese writing system was imported into Japan, and thus is a fairly ancient word. The definition is intended to be of more generic use rather than in reference to rope bondage, but it has been used as such, most notably by Ito Seiu, since the 1950s. *Kinbaku* is a new word (most likely started being used during the twentieth century) created by combining two Chinese characters that mean "in a tight way" and "to tie securely."[34] Looking more closely at the definitions of the words, shibari means simply to tie, but kinbaku indicates tying tightly to the point of restraint or immobility. Despite these semantic differences, in terms of contemporary usage, these terms are becoming interchangeable. Clearly, this creates a great deal of confusion and is the source of never-ending debate within the bondage community.

For the purposes of simplicity, this chapter will differentiate the two schools according to the most popular opinion—that

---

32 Ibid.

33 Kirigami, "Shibari VS Kinbaku," *Rope Tales* (blog), accessed November 20, 2017, https://www.ropetales.com/shibari-vs-kinbaku/.

34 Ibid.

shibari simply refers to the art of tying, whereas kinbaku implies a strong emotional exchange between the Top and bottom through the medium of the rope. No matter which word is used in reference to a bondage activity, both use patterns derived from *Hojo-jutsu* ties that have been significantly modified to make them safer and more comfortable for erotic purposes. This development of rope from a device of subjugation and torture to an art form that touts comfort, safety, and connection is a beautiful transformation that highlights the democratizing nature of engaging in consensual bondage.

The community has never been as vibrant as it is today. While YouTube tutorials and BDSM education sites have made accessing knowledge about tying rope much easier, it is advisable that you do as much hands-on learning as possible. Don't get me wrong, working through the tutorials from this book or the aforementioned sites is an important part of your learning process. That being said, there are many instances where immediate feedback from an expert would be helpful. Just as meeting fitness goals is more likely when working at a gym with a trainer rather than at home with a workout video, learning to use rope bondage safely and effectively is best done with supervision and guidance. To provide opportunities for this, conventions are held at hotels where novices can stay with bondage experts for the weekend while garnering as many bondage tips and experiences as they are able to. There are also smaller skill-share events called "Rope Bites" that are hosted in cities all around the United States and even internationally. You can find more information about those at www.ropebite.com.

## Advanced Thoughts on Japanese Rope Bondage

As we discussed in Section 1, there are a myriad of motivations for engaging in bondage activities. One interesting perspective about restraint that shares roots in Japanese culture is a phenomenon referred to as *urami*, which explores the ability of restraint to dislodge feelings and memories that have been buried deep and help them float to the surface.[35] Urami is built upon the concept of *ura*, that which is kept concealed or hidden, as opposed to *omote*, which means outside or visible on the surface. Thoughts, feelings, and desires that arise but are kept private are referred to as *omoi*. On a more spiritual level, urami comes from the "Shinto/Buddhist idea where the soul is bound to Earth by unfulfilled desires. These desires can be anything—unrequited love, unexpressed gratitude, unfinished business."[36]

Specifically in Japanese culture (but also reflected in a variety of cultures around the globe) the separation of the public and private selves is important. We frequently find ourselves wearing figurative masks in order to comply with states of being that are deemed acceptable by authority figures. Restricting someone's freedom of movement by introducing the element of restraint creates the context for feelings of resentment (urami) toward authority figures to arise. Generally conflated with these feelings of resentment toward authority is the omoi (unfulfilled desire), though in the context of erotic bondage, the authority figure is usually a trusted and beloved partner. It is important to note that in this context, the urami is not anger or resentment directed at the bondage Top, but instead is an internal struggle that allows the personal and private self to be revealed. Therefore, practitioners usually find that once the feelings have been activated

---

35 "Itoh Seiu: Urami and the Drama of Rope," *Kinbaku Today* (blog), December 19, 2016, http://www.kinbakutoday.com/itoh-seiu-urami-drama-rope/.

36 Zack Davisson, "The History of Hausu." *Henry Art Gallery* (blog), January 2, 2014, https://hankblog.wordpress.com/2014/01/02/the-history-of-hausu/.

or released, the context of a scene actually opens up the omoi (unfulfilled desire) and gives it space for expression. For this reason, many people choose to use restraint as a way to "dance with their demons" or engage with their shadow sides and work through trauma, either on their own or with loved ones.

The artwork of Sensei Ito Seiu is revered as containing the best depictions of urami and drama that rope bondage has to offer. If you're confused or curious about what this process looks like, I would recommend delving into his work. I would also recommend, all jargon aside, that you take a moment to think about your daily struggles—the struggles that you keep to yourself, the resentments that are buried deep down and only peek out during times of crisis, and the grudges that you don't even remember that you're holding. For a moment, let all of those feelings bubble up inside you. Now imagine the gravity of the cathartic release that sharing these feelings with a loved one without judgment would provide. It seems like a beautiful, heart-swelling experience, right? Ultimately, the concept of urami is a concept of deep connection and emotional processing.

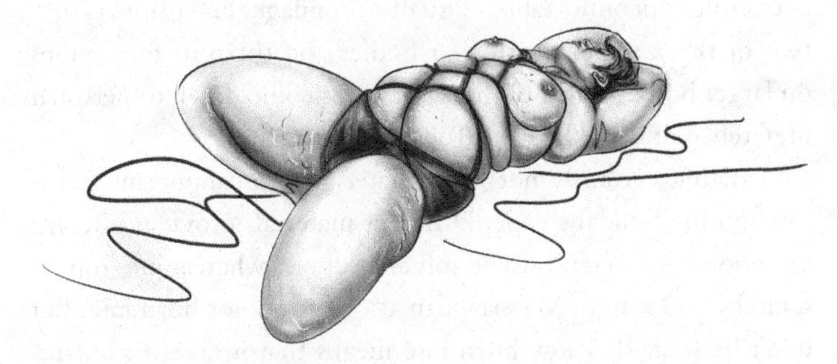

## Selecting your rope

Now that you've been briefed on the history of Japanese rope bondage, as well as the concept of urami, you must be itching to get your hands on some rope!

To start, you'll want to determine what length of rope to

use. Most riggers determine this by their arm span, and what seems manageable to handle without getting tangled. While it's possible to join two lengths of rope, it's less of a hassle to have the proper length that you need in the first place. It is also more aesthetically pleasing if you don't have any knots showing where the ropes were joined. The standard length for restrictive ties is usually around twenty-five to thirty feet. However, if you're planning on tying an elaborate pattern, or you'll be regularly tying up a plus-size partner, you may choose to go with up to fifty feet. The longer the rope gets, the more difficult it is to manage, so it's recommended that you do not use rope lengths over fifty feet.

Thickness is another important aspect of bondage rope. The thickness of rope can determine which body parts it should be used on and also how much it cuts into the flesh. Thinner ropes tend to be good for genital bondage or microbondage on the face or fingers, but are uncomfortable for restraint. The number of wraps also determines how much the rope cuts into the flesh. The more wraps, the more weight the rope can hold without becoming uncomfortable. Usually, bondage practitioners use two or three wraps on smaller bodies and three to four wraps on larger bodies. Most of these decisions come down to personal preference of both the rope Top and bottom.

Last but certainly not least, material is an important factor in choosing bondage rope. Different materials provide different sensations: nylon tends to be soft and supple, whereas jute rope is scratchy and rough. Material can also account for burn rate, but don't be fooled! A low burn rate means that it takes little friction to cause a rope burn, whereas a high burn rate means that it is more difficult to cause a rope burn. As you probably know from your days on the playground or rock climbing, rope burns can be nasty, so make sure that you're paying attention to the material of the rope that you're using before drawing it across someone's skin. Each different material also has different safety and cleaning considerations.

### *Types of Rope*[37]

**Synthetic rope:** Synthetic rope is wonderful for beginner rope-bondage practitioners. It is the most affordable type of rope, so it's great for beginners who aren't sure that they're ready to invest $300 to $500 on a rope kit (yes, they do get that expensive!). Synthetic materials are hypoallergenic, easy to clean, and low maintenance. Despite all of their wonderful qualities, synthetic ropes have a low burn rate, which means they can cause rope burns easily. It is often suggested to keep two or three fingers between the rope and skin when dragging it quickly to avoid such burns.

**Nylon:** Nylon rope comes in a variety of beautiful colors and is machine washable, making it great for body harnesses, crotch ropes, or decorative ties. It can be used for load bearing, but due to the stretch, this requires advanced technique.

**Hempex:** Hempex is faux-hemp rope. It is a great choice for people who would like to emulate the look of natural fiber rope but avoid the high cost or extensive maintenance. It's both easily washable and dryable and incredibly durable. Hempex rope does tend to appear fuzzy with heavy use and multiple washings, but it retains its strength. The drawbacks are purely aesthetic.

**Natural fiber rope:** Natural fiber rope is popular among experienced bondage practitioners and "riggers" who like to do load-bearing ties due to its strength and the fact that it doesn't stretch easily. It also has a very high burn rate, so it's less likely you'll

---

37 "Rope Selection," Knot Right Supply LLC, 2016, http://www.knotrightsupply.com/info/rope-selection/.

give your partner rope burns when pulling it across their skin. In rope making, the same fiber can be used to create a variety of styles of rope, which means that natural fibers are easily customizable to the specifications that each rigger prefers.

One setback with natural fiber ropes is that they wear out. Most regular bondage practitioners will replace their suspension rope kits every six to twelve months, but this varies based on how often the ropes are used, and for what purpose. The more stress you regularly put on the rope, the faster it will wear out. These ropes also require regular conditioning. That might include working, oiling, singeing, waxing, or whipping, to name a few techniques. Therefore, rope-maintenance knowledge is also required. With the exception of cotton rope, they are also harder to wash because they need to be dried under tension to prevent shrinkage, usually meaning that if a partner's bodily fluids come in contact with the rope, that rope is only ever used on that one play partner.

**Cotton:** Often marketed as clothesline, cotton rope can be found easily and priced very cheaply. Its price, availability, and ease of tying makes it great for beginners. Easy to clean and wash, cotton rope is recommended primarily for genital bondage and crotch ropes.

**Silk/bamboo:** Silk and bamboo ropes are considered to be luxury ropes due to the comfort that they provide and their expense. Bamboo has less grip than cotton or silk rope, but it has natural antibacterial properties and a very smooth, soft feel against the skin. It is best used for decorative ties, or restrictive ties with well-behaved bottoms. Silk rope has a slightly better grip and can be used for both decorative and restrictive ties with partners who prioritize comfort.

**Hemp/jute:** Very popular with experienced riggers, these fibers have great grip and are very easy to tie with. Jute is smoother and lighter than hemp and compresses more easily. This can make load-bearing ties hard to untie for the inexperienced rigger. Another important factor with natural fiber rope made from grasses and plants is that it might trigger allergies for those with grass/hay fever allergies.

**Coconut:** Coconut rope doesn't need too much maintenance. It is incredibly scratchy and rough—wonderful for people who enjoy pain play with their rope. It does lose fibers that can produce nasty splinters if they get under the skin, so be sure to have tweezers handy.

## TUTORIALS

Below you will find tutorials that invoke traditional Japanese patterns with the use of rope as a binding material, which should serve as the base of your bondage foundation. Later in the book, you will see the same patterns reappear, but with less-traditional tools and applications.

### 1. Single-Column Tie

1.1 Make a bight in the rope by folding it in half. The bight is the loop that the middle section of the rope makes when folded. The other end of the rope is called the running end.

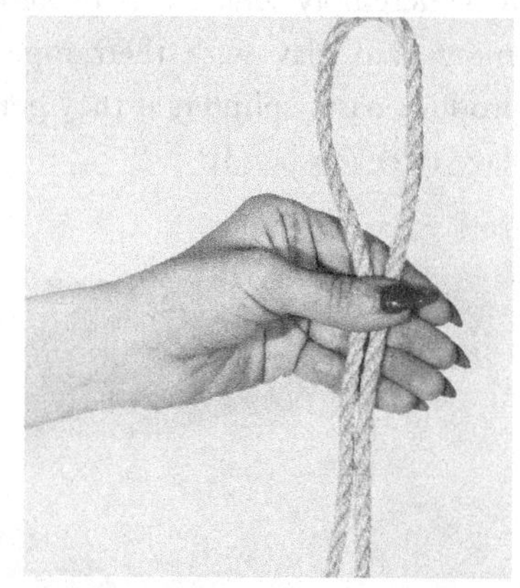

1.2 Place the bight on limb/column, positioned so that the rope can wrap from the side of the appendage closest to the body toward the end of the limb.

1.3 Wrap around the limb/column three or four times, leaving space for one or two fingers underneath the rope (this is important for comfort and circulation).

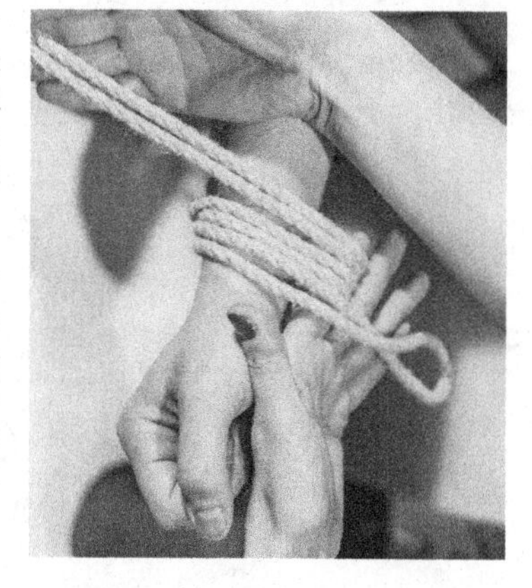

1.4 Twist the rope ends to trade sides/directions.

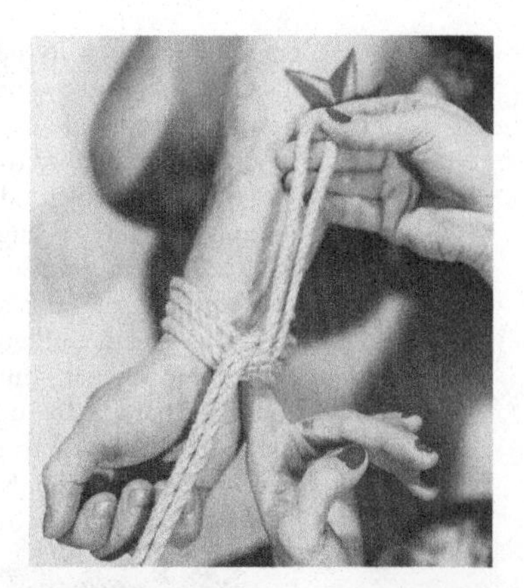

1.5 Tie off the ends with a knot of your choice. In this tutorial, we used the Somerville bowline knot. Watch our video tutorial at the Cleis Press YouTube channel to learn how to tie a Somerville bowline knot.

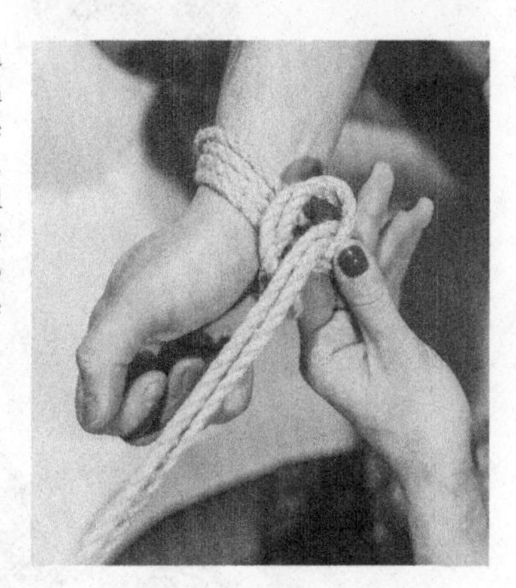

1.5.1 For readers without access to the video tutorial: Loop the running end around the bight end to create a circle, with an X at the bottom where the running end crosses over itself. Pass the bight end over the X, underneath all of the wraps, and back up through the loop created by the running end (you can grab it with your fingers from above and pull it up through the loop for more ease). Finally, tighten the knot by tugging on the bight end, then the running end, and pushing the sides of the knot in toward the center. Once the knot is well formed, tighten it down more by pushing everything together. Now what you will have is a knot/cuff that will not collapse, and that can be untied very quickly in the case of an emergency. Note: If you use the loop that is left as an attachment point, or run the running ends through the loop before tying it off, the knot will take longer to untie, so be mindful of that.

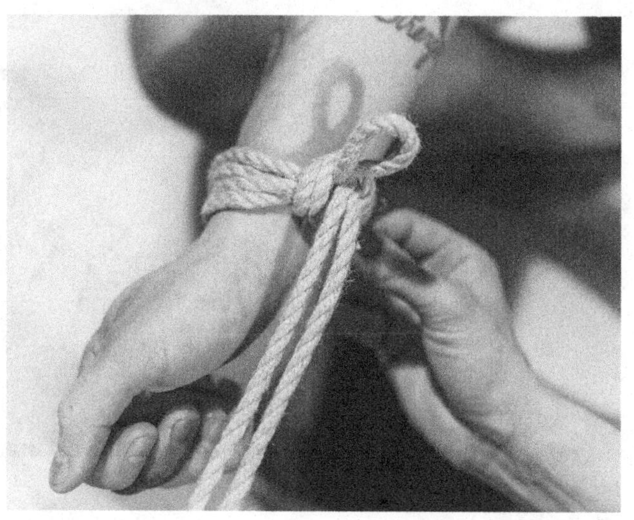

*Top: Mildred S. Pierce. Bottom: Gage*

## 2. Double-Column Tie

2.1 Follow steps 1.1-1.3, this time around two limbs.

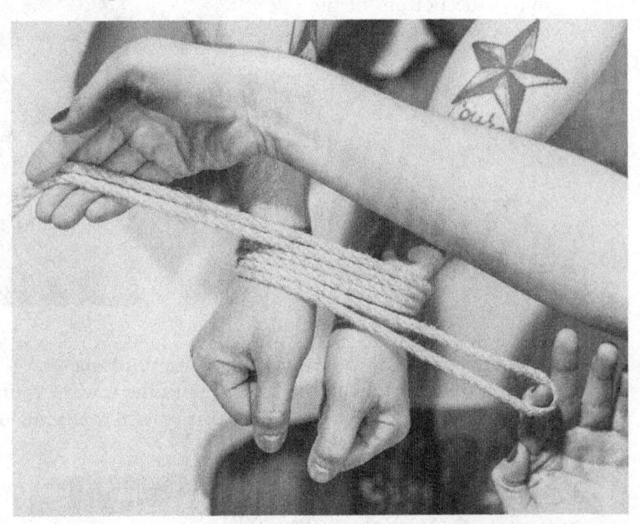

2.2 Twist the ends to change the directions of each rope. One end should be pointing toward you and one should be pointing toward your bottom's body.

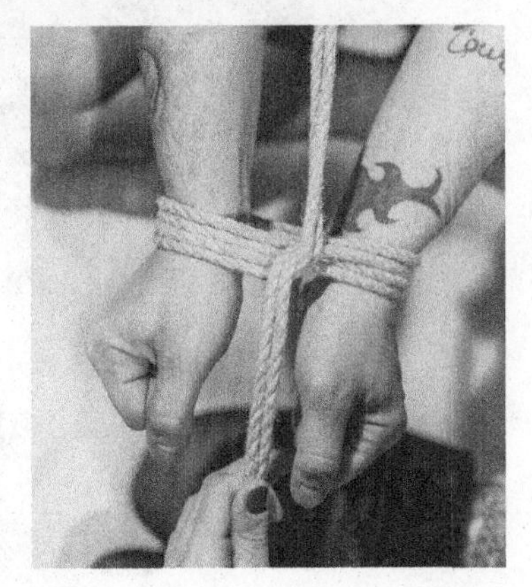

2.3 Move ropes down between the tied limbs on the horizontal axis, around the bottom of the wraps you've made.

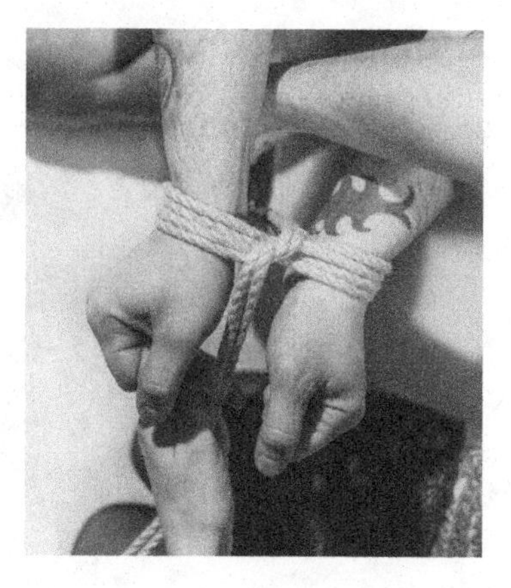

2.4 Twist the rope ends to change directions, until one end is again pointing toward you and the other is pointing toward your partner, this time underneath the wraps. Bring both rope ends around the wraps and back up to the top.

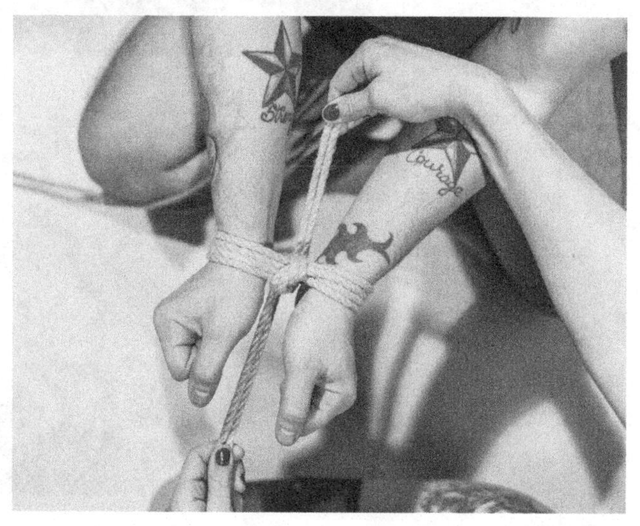

2.5 Once the rope ends are back up to the top, tie them off with a knot of your choice. We used the Somerville bowline again here (see 1.5 on page 73).

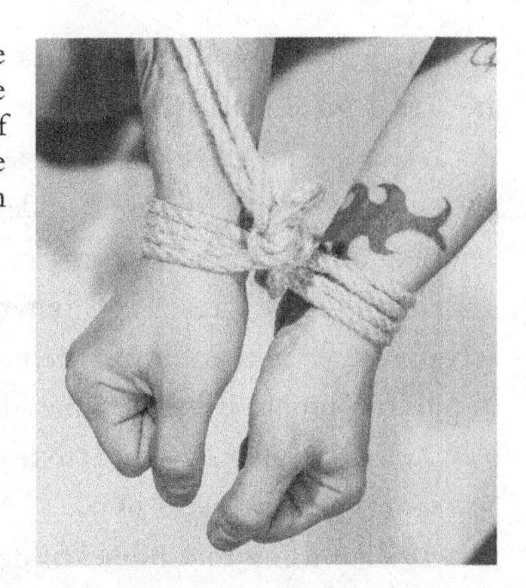

2.6 Tie off any way you'd like, either to an anchor point or to a harness.

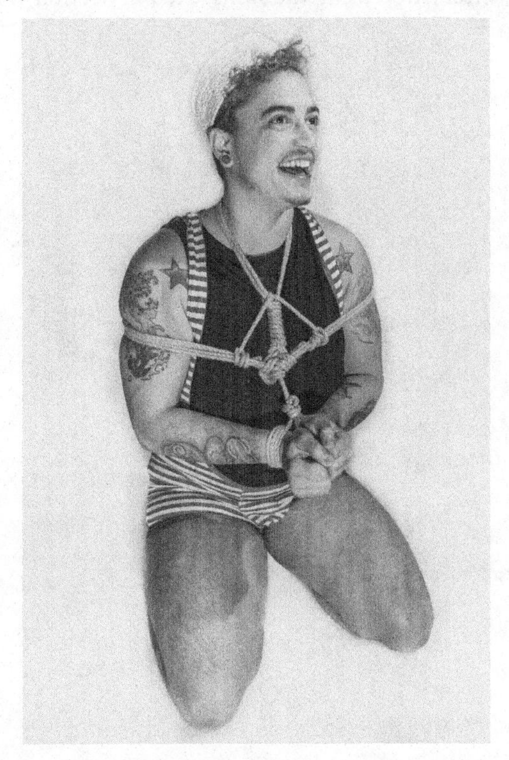

*Top: Mildred S. Pierce. Bottom: Gage.*

**Safety precautions:** It's important to note that these variations are based on shibari ties, not the Japanese patterns themselves. Because rope bondage is very tricky to convey in writing and photographs, the patterns included here are at the most basic level and include knots that are functional but that might collapse under substantial pressure if not tied correctly. Take this into account when you are using them, and inform your partner not to pull too much. It is recommended that you attend a live class or watch some video tutorials to learn about noncollapsible knots and more intricate patterns.

If you're using the single- or double-column ties around the wrists, be sure not to ratchet them down too tightly. Check in on circulation using the skills listed in Section 1.

## Other Examples of Japanese Rope Bondage

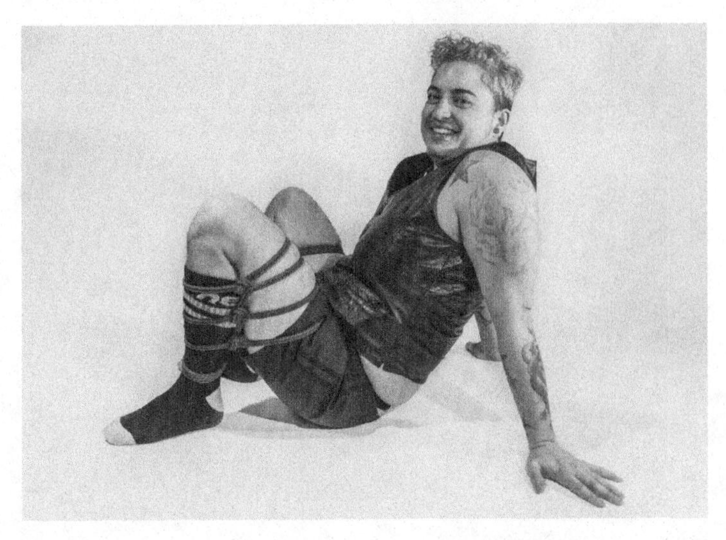

*Bent Leg Tie (Futomomo). Bottom: Gage. Top: Oz.*

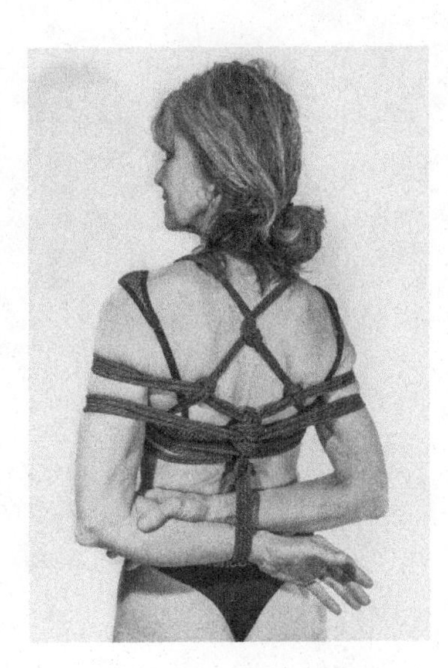

*Takate-Kote (Box Tie).*
*Bottom: Simone. Top: Oz.*

CHAPTER

4

# DEVICE BONDAGE

As you read in the previous chapter, rope has evolved from a traditional Japanese restraint device into an art form with a variety of applications. Outside of rope, there are myriad other bondage devices that have been invented for the purposes of not just restraint, but also erotic stimulation, control, and torture. Many of these devices are easy to acquire, come prefabricated, and are fairly intuitive to use. Whereas it might take years to master rope skills enough to produce a sound box tie, securing someone's arms behind their back using handcuffs or cuffs and carabiners only takes a few minutes. Other devices are homemade, dreamed up by mad-scientist types who enjoy experimenting with construction and design. If you are one of those people, be sure to check out Kink.com's aptly named porn channel, "Device Bondage," for ideas.

We will begin this chapter by exploring the invention and evolution of one of the most essential bondage devices, the key. Then we will continue our exploration through some of the many restraint bondage devices that exist today, as well as devices intended for erotic stimulation, control, and torture.

## Keys

Locks and keys are tools that are used to provide security and control who can access things like your car, post office box, and the front door to your home. Your key ring might be expanding soon, as many bondage devices like handcuffs and shackles use locks and keys for the same reasons. The oldest example of a lock and key device was found in the ruins of an area that was once called Nineveh (modern-day Mosul, Iraq).[38] "The area was settled as early as 6000 BCE, and by 3000, had become an important religious center for worship of the goddess Ishtar."[39] Ishtar is also known as Goddess Inanna, the matriarch of modern Dominatrix culture. Ancient cuneiform texts consisting of hymns to Inanna depict her as a powerful sexual female who dominated men and gods alike,[40] so it is fitting that keys, one of the ultimate symbols of bondage, were created in her region.

During the Middle Ages, most developed cities were surrounded by high walls and fortresses. These walls were boundaries set by rulers in order to keep unpredictable wildlife and enemies out, and were only able to be opened by those deemed worthy enough to guard the city gate. Thus, it became a gesture of trust and goodwill to present visiting dignitaries with a key to the city.[41] Despite the lack of border walls around most cities today, the gesture of presenting keys is still similar symbolically and is used frequently to honor visitors. Within the culture of BDSM, presenting a Dominant with the keys to one's

---

38 "History of Keys—Who Invented Keys?," *History of Keys* (blog), 2018, accessed December 1, 2017, http://www.historyofkeys.com/keys-history/history-of-keys/.

39 Ancient History Encyclopedia, s.v. "Nineveh," by Joshua J. Mark, March 6, 2011, https://www.ancient.eu/nineveh/.

40 Anne O. Nomis, *The History and Arts of the Dominatrix* (Mary Egan Publishing & Anna Nomis Ltd., 2013), 53.

41 Stacy Conradt, "Does the Key to the City Actually Open Anything?" *Mental Floss* (blog), May 13, 2012, http://mentalfloss.com/article/30744/does-key-city-actually-open-anything.

chastity device is comparable to this ancient tradition. Rather than presenting keys to a city, a submissive in chastity presents the keys to their orgasm, a sacred privilege.

Throughout the ages, locks and keys have been developed into highly intricate security systems. The advancements of engineering during the Industrial Revolution led to the creation of highly complex locks that were difficult to pick or bypass. In an effort to thwart the skeleton key (a key that could open almost any lock), and lock pickers, inventor Joseph Bramah created the "Challenge Lock." Sources disagree on the exact dates, but somewhere between 1784 and 1801, Bramah opened a shop, Bramah Lock Company, and displayed the Challenge Lock in the window. He proposed that whomever could defeat the challenge by picking or opening the lock would be rewarded with two hundred gold guineas (approximately $200-300 in today's currency, and a great fortune in that era). The lock remained unpicked for years until, at the Great Exhibition of 1851, American locksmith Alfred C. Hobbs figured it out. It took him fifty-one hours to solve the puzzle, demonstrating just how advanced the technology had become.[42]

Many locks today are still variants of Bramah's original designs. A major design flaw of keys that has not been completely solved is that if they are lost or misplaced, there is little one can do to open the lock, unless they have fifty-one hours to spare like Alfred Hobbs did. For this reason, having contingency plans like obtaining copies of keys, using bolt cutters, or having a kinky locksmith on hand are very important. In self-bondage scenarios or situations wherein a submissive is locked into a device by their Dominant, sealing a copy key in wax or ice are great contingency plans.

---

42 Adam Clark Estes, "The History and Future of Locks and Keys," *Gizmodo* (blog), October 20, 2015, https://gizmodo.com/the-history-and-future-of-locks-and-keys-1735694812.

Locks and keys are only one example of tools that have been created with the purpose of utility for bondage and restraint. There are a wide variety of restraint devices used in modern-day bondage scenes.

## Device Bondage: Restraint

As you learned in the chapter about Japanese rope bondage, restraint is undeniably the primary objective of most bondage activities. This doesn't exclude restrictive bondage from looking nice, and in fact, lots of restrictive bondage is beautiful to look at. The catch is that if the bondage looks pretty but is easily escapable, a bottom who is looking for a sensation of captivity is not going to be satisfied. For this reason, restrictive bondage must be strong and escape-proof. Below you will find the descriptions of a variety of bondage devices that can reliably be used for restraint.

**Cuffs[43]:** Cuffs are easy to use and durable, two qualities that make them a great go-to toy for practitioners of every level. Whether you're a pillow princess who prefers comfortably fuzzy cuffs or a prisoner who craves cold metal, a bondage novice or experienced practitioner, these devices are for you.

**Beginner cuffs:** The most important quality of a beginner cuff is that it is easy to use. Cuffs with snaps, zippers, or Velcro straps are easy to operate and allow for quick capture and release. They also make for easy escape, so make sure that if you're using beginner cuffs, you have a willing "victim." Inexpensive yet reliable materials such as neoprene or faux fur are generally used for these types of cuffs. Because these materials are durable but not load tested, they should only be used for basic restraint and floor-

---

43 "How to Choose Handcuffs," *How-To and Guides* (blog), Secret Pleasures Boutique, accessed November 3, 2017, http://www.secretpleasuresboutique.com/How-To-Choose-Handcuffs_c_111.html.

work, and not for any load-bearing activities. When equipped with rings—often called D-rings because they are shaped like an uppercase D—cuffs can be used to bind your partner to furniture. They can also be used in conjunction with other bondage gear, such as spreader bars.

**Intermediate cuffs:** Intermediate cuffs provide a bit more security than beginner cuffs. They're harder to put on and harder to struggle out of or take off. The two main types of intermediate cuffs are leather and metal cuffs. Leather cuffs are both durable and dynamic, which is why they serve as a great intermediate cuff. Leather is pricey and requires cleaning and conditioning, which makes it a more difficult material to care for, but if maintained properly, a single pair of cuffs can last over twenty-five years! Some leather cuffs are lined with fabric or fur to make them more comfortable for long-term wear. Things that clean leather might ruin fabric and fur and vice versa, so these types of cuffs require even more careful upkeep.

Like leather cuffs, metal handcuffs are durable and highly effective. They're also more risky than leather or neoprene, so be careful. The hard metal can be psychologically effective, but uncomfortable, and it increases the risk of nerve damage or injury if pressure is placed on the cuff. The metal tends to chafe skin and hit delicate bones in the wrists or ankles. This makes handcuffs a poor option for any sort of scenario where struggle/squirming will be involved. If you must struggle, keep in mind that single-locking cuffs act like a slipknot and can tighten at any time, so you should not use them. Instead, you should use police-style double-locking cuffs, which are equipped with a lock that prevents them from closing all the way, and will maintain the level of tightness at which they are originally set. That being said, handcuffs are best utilized in bondage scenes where the cuffed limbs can be at rest while secured to the bedpost.

The most challenging aspect of handcuffs is that they can only be removed with a key once they are locked. If the key is lost, the only way to free someone without embarrassment is a bolt cutter or expert lock picker. In that regard, they are great for bottoms who consider themselves to be escape artists.

**Advanced cuffs:** Wraparound cuffs (also called suspension cuffs) are wonderful for squirmy bottoms who love the power dynamics of struggle and resistance. As you read in the safety section in Chapter 2, pulling or straining against cuffs has the potential to cause nerve damage or impair circulation. Wraparound cuffs mitigate that issue by using wider bands that bolster the wearer's wrists in order to better support the weight of their body. A grip cuff is a modified style that employs a handle. These cuffs can support the entire weight of the bottom; in fact they can be used to completely suspend someone off the ground. Hanging suspended by the wrists does put tension on the chest cavity, making it difficult to breathe, so frequent check-ins are required. Please note that this is not intended to be an explanation of how to suspend a bottom safely. Suspension bondage is an advanced technique that requires in-person instruction.

### *Hardware*[44]

**Panic snaps:** Panic snaps are aptly named, as they're meant to be used when release is needed immediately. The devices are easy to unsnap with one hand no matter how much weight is on them, making quick release a snap!

**Double-ended snap hook:** Double-ended snap hooks have a clip at each end, making them a quick way to attach a set of cuffs to other equipment, including straps, chains, D-rings, furniture,

---

44 Ibid.

and more. They do not lock and are fairly easy to use in quick-release scenarios, but can become jammed if carrying a weight load.

**Carabiners:** Often used for rock climbing, carabiners are a sturdy and versatile tool for fastening restraints. They come in locking and nonlocking styles, depending on how quickly they need to be removed. Carabiners are often weight tested for heavy load bearing and are commonly used in suspension bondage. They're also great for attaching rope or impact toys to your belt loop for quick access!

### *Furniture*

The St. Andrew's cross and the spanking bench are the most common pieces of BDSM furniture. While there are companies that make discreet versions of these items that fold up to go under the bed, they are usually considerable financial investments, and therefore BDSM furniture is most often found at commercial dungeons and places where they can be displayed out in the open.

St. Andrew's crosses typically provide restraining points for the wrists, ankles, and waist, leaving the bottom in a very exposed yet supported spread-eagle position. Being restrained facing the cross leaves the bottom's backside accessible for impact play like spanking or whipping, whereas being restrained with one's back to the cross leaves the bottom vulnerable to sexual teasing. It is important to check in frequently when someone is tied to a St. Andrew's cross, as their arms are secured above the head, which can become uncomfortable or lead to dizziness.

A spanking bench is a piece of furniture that is used to position the bottom for a spanking scene. While there are many styles and sizes, the most popular spanking bench is a sawhorse with a padded top and rests for the knees. Similar to the St. Andrew's cross, it is possible for bottoms to be lashed to this piece of furniture in order to receive impact play or sexual teasing. Due to the fact that the bottom can lie on their stomach, this piece of furniture is more comfortable and accessible than the St. Andrew's cross, and can be used for longer periods of play.

### *Other Restraint Devices*

**Restraint systems:** Restraint systems are wonderful for novice bondage practitioners who have not yet mastered the skills of rope bondage. They consist of multiple items that are meant to be used together as a set and can be purchased as a single kit. For instance, an under-the-bed restraint system consists of elastic straps that wrap around your mattress, with modifiable straps and cuffs. They provide easy and effective solutions for restraining a partner in a variety of positions, including the hogtie, spread eagle, and box tie, that can be applied and removed quickly. Typically restraint systems are made from a combination of nylon, neoprene, leather, and/or metal.

**Spreader bar:** Spreader bars have been popular bondage devices for years but recently experienced a spike in sales due to their popularization by the *Fifty Shades of Grey* series. Objectifying in addition to practical, a spreader bar holds the legs or arms apart, allowing unrevokable access to the Top. Spreader bars are typically made out of metal or bamboo, with built-in attachment points on each end. It is recommended that when used on a standing bottom, a spreader bar be used in conjunction with grip cuffs for the wrists, as having the legs spread in a wide position can throw off balance.

**Straitjackets:** Straitjackets are a wonderful example of the confluence of a variety of types of bondage into one very practical tool. They are garments, and therefore technically costume bondage, but the arms are secured behind the back to restrain people who might cause harm to themselves or others. Originally an instrument of restraint from the Victorian era of medicine, straitjackets were used to prevent those with mental illness from inflicting harm on themselves or others, even when they were not attended by a doctor. Eventually they became an item of intrigue for escapologists and magicians. Wearing a straitjacket for long periods of time might cause pain for the wearer. Due to the bent position of the elbows, blood flow to the ulnar nerves becomes limited, which can cause swelling.[45] Other safety concerns for straightjackets include numbness or tingling due to disrupted circulation, and pain caused by muscle stiffness after being restrained in the same position for a long period of time. Hospitals and mental health facilities are required to conform to strict monitoring protocols when outfitting people in straitjackets, and you should, too. In consensual BDSM settings, straitjackets are best implemented with bottoms who desire a medical-themed scene or who consider themselves to enjoy struggle or escapology.

### *Some Tips for Restraint*

One of the most challenging objectives within restrictive bondage is immobilizing the bottom enough while leaving the skin or other body parts accessible to the Top. Cuff restraints attached to furniture will restrict movement of the limbs but not of the head, fingers or toes. Mental bondage or training does come into play here, as it teaches the bottom to use the restraint as a reminder to hold still (we will explore mental bondage in depth in the next chapter). If the play is going to venture into pain or pleasure exploration, the bottom will likely need the security and support

---

45 Ed Zimney, MD, "Cell Phone Elbow Isn't Always Due to Cell Phone Use," *Personal Takes* (blog), *Everyday Health*, June 4, 2009, https://www.everydayhealth.com/columns/zimney-health-and-medical-news-you-can-use/cell-phone-elbow-isnt-always-due-to-cell-phone-use/.

of structurally sound bondage as well as something to pull on or thrash around within. In this light, placing a bottom in restrictive bondage can be seen as an act of mercy.

## Erotic Stimulation and Control

It's time to move on to other uses for bondage, beyond restraint. What better place to start than with erotic stimulation and control? As you can probably imagine, bondage sex is incredibly erotic. The ways in which bondage devices can be used to stimulate or starve the erogenous zones are vast. Friction from rope or leather alone can produce orgasm, but one of the most common applications of bondage for erotic stimulation is the direction or restriction of blood flow to the genitals. Conversely, utilizing chastity devices or plugs to keep the genital regions "on lockdown" are torturously effective methods of erotic bondage.

### *Erotic Stimulation*

> *"That which we call a rose by any other name would smell as sweet."*
>
> —William Shakespeare[46]

A note on gender, sex, and genitalia: No matter how you identify, you have the right to refer to your genitals as you see fit. Some people call them "bits" or make up other slang terms to refer to them, and other people call them by their anatomical names. Unfortunately, anatomical names for genitalia refer to sex rather than gender. For those who do not ascribe to the gender binary, using gendered names for genitalia can cause feelings of dysphoria. I know plenty of people who were assigned male at birth who refer to their genitalia as their "clit" and

46 William Shakespeare, *Romeo and Juliet,* ed. Craig, W.J. (London: Oxford University Press, 2000), 2.2.47-48.

"ovaries" or people who were assigned female at birth who use the word "cock" to describe what is between their legs. In order to minimize confusion for beginners while being respectful to nonbinary folks, this chapter and all subsequent chapters that discuss genitalia will refer to devices with their widely accepted gendered names, but will attempt to discuss their applications with gender-neutral language.

**Suction cups:** Suction pumps (often called "cock pumps") and suction cups (often called "nipple suction cups") are designed to increase sensitivity in an erogenous zone. Although they are named for specific body parts, pumps and cups work great on almost any fleshy body part as long as body hair is removed and the device can make a seal against the skin. By creating a vacuum seal, pumps and cups increase circulation and then trap the blood within the erogenous zone until the seal is released. It is this trapping of the blood that qualifies suction cups as bondage devices, though many people consider them to be sensation toys.

**Cock rings:** Cock rings are great for people with bio-dicks and similarly protruding genitalia. Wearing one restricts the flow of blood out of an erection, often causing it to become harder, more tumescent, and more sensitive and last for a longer period of time. They come in a wide variety of styles including rubber, rope, metal, silicone, and even vibrating models.

**Crotch rope:** Known as *sakura* or "cherry blossom" in Japanese rope bondage, the crotch rope is a technique that involves passing the rope through the legs to apply pressure to the genitals. For those folks who have a highly sensitive mound of nerve endings between their legs, carefully placing knots that will rub against it is a favorite practice. Folks with protruding genitalia will likely need to split the ropes and provide a hole for the genitalia to pass through in order to avoid obstructing the bondage or bending the genitalia in an uncomfortable manner.

No matter how the rope conforms to your genitals, wearing crotch rope is an extremely erotic experience. Ito Seiu reportedly said that, when released, the tie should feel like the "ethereal moment at which a cherry blossom falls from the tree." Anyone who has worn crotch rope will tell you that being released from it offers much more relief than watching the beauty of nature! Wearing crotch rope is quite the intense experience, but it is this intensity that makes it so popular. Rope carries vibration very strongly, so adding a vibrator into the mix by placing it up close to the rope amps the whole predicament up another level! Because the rope passes through the legs, restricting access to the genitals and anus, it is used most commonly as a part of tease and denial.

**CBT rope:** The moniker "cock and ball torture," or CBT, is traditionally used in BDSM to refer to activities that inflict pain upon protruding genitalia. As such genitalia are not only easy to wrap in rope, but hypersensitive to a variety of pleasurable and painful sensations, a whole discipline of rope bondage has arisen devoted specifically to the use of rope to bind, tease, and torture such genitalia. Techniques often involve the use of thin twine, to better grip and inflict sensation on tender, squirmy bits.

### *Erotic Control*

**Chastity devices:** A chastity device is a bondage tool that can be worn to prevent the wearer from having intercourse or participating in any other sexual activities like oral sex and manual stimulation. Submissive partners typically wear these devices as a means to relinquish control of their sexual freedoms to their Dominant partners. Chastity devices are often secured with a small padlock, to which the Dominant holds the key. They can also be secured with numbered plastic tags, for easy removal in an emergency when the Dominant is not present. There are chastity devices for all types of genitals, so shopping around for the right size and fit are important. They are advanced-level bondage tools, and should be researched heavily and eased into slowly.

**Plugs:** Plugs are generally used for sexual pleasure and to dilate the anus, vagina, or urethra for sexual purposes. They provide a great deal of sensation, which people often describe as "full." The fullness, in conjunction with some added features, turns plugs into another way of controlling and preventing sexual activity. Urethral plugs with a collar can be worn as jewelry, not allowing anything (particularly ejaculate) to pass through the hole. When attached to locking belts or piercings, a plug can be used as a chastity device. With the simple turn of a key, locking anal plugs can spread open wide and lock into place. With plugs, the possibilities are vast, just like the opening in your bottom will feel. Like any other training device, they should be introduced incrementally in size and duration to avoid injury and discomfort. Because these items are being inserted into body cavities, they should all be sterilized beforehand, and should be inserted gently and without great force to avoid injury.

**Cock and ball devices:** A variation on cock rings, cock and ball devices are best used on bio-cocks, testicles, and similarly protruding genitalia. They are meant to be used to stretch the balls away from the body in a manner that is both pleasurable and frustrating. Achieving orgasm while the balls are tied can be quite painful, depending on one's anatomy and how far from the body the scrotum is stretched. Because the balls generally retract into the body when orgasming, a band around the testicles can be used as a deterrent for orgasm. Using ball stretchers can permanently elongate the scrotum, so make sure your partner is aware of this before engaging in it regularly. It is imperative that you are very careful with cock and ball devices. If they are too tight, they can cut off blood circulation and cause permanent damage. Wearing stretchers that are too long or heavy can damage the delicate tissues in the scrotum or crush the testicles. If things start to feel cold or turn blue, remove the bondage immediately. That being said, if done correctly, the sensation and effects of ball bondage are fantastic. Go slow, build it up incrementally, and make sure that your partner is communicating to you about how it feels.

## Torture

Certain bondage devices are built for the specific purpose of causing pain. Throughout human history, a variety of cultures have ascribed to the idea that only through pain and suffering can a person achieve innocence after they commit a sin. This widely proliferated belief system predicated the creation of some of the planet's cruelest torture devices, some of which have been modified for safe use within the context of BDSM relationships.

**Scold's bridle:** During the Middle Ages, "scold" was a pejorative term used to describe a woman who was constantly displeased or nagging too much. During this time, women were still seen as property, and as such expected to be docile and obedient. The scold's bridle was invented to humiliate women in an effort to deter them from speaking out of turn. In a system that mirrors modern-day wealth disparity in many ways, the scold's bridle was exclusively applied to women of the lower social class, while members of the court were permitted to gossip and jest without the fear of being punished.

If accused of scolding, a woman would be fitted with the iron framework system and forced to don it like a mask. The bridle bit, a small piece of metal, would be placed in the woman's mouth and pressed onto the tongue to prevent her from talking. Sometimes a spike that would gouge the tongue with any movement was attached to the bridle bit, discouraging its victim from speaking.[47] Similar to the tradition of public humiliation in Japanese rope bondage, the wearer of a scold's bridle would be marched through town at the end a leash carried by her husband or another male authority figure. German versions of the scold's bridle were affixed with a bell in order to attract more attention during this walk of shame.

**Heretic's fork:** Another tongue-tying torture device of the Middle Ages was the heretic's fork. This device consisted of a length of metal with pointed, forked metal tips on each end. Placed between the breastbone and the throat, and secured with a leather strap around the neck, the heretic's fork was intended to impale blasphemers, liars, or people who spoke the Lord's name in vain. The punishment made it nearly impossible for its victims to speak or sleep. The moment their jaw opened or their head dropped with fatigue, the prongs pierced their throat or chest, causing great pain. While wearing the device, even swallowing became torturous—"the strap compresses the Adam's apple, inducing brief spasms of suffocation."[48] The imposed period of silence in conjunction with painful torture and sleep deprivation was believed to encourage confessions from the victims, and proved to be successful at doing so.

In today's BDSM culture, while modified versions of scold's bridles and heretic's forks are occasionally spotted in the dungeon,

---

47 Brad Smithfield, "Scold's bridle—The gruesome medieval torture instrument worn to deter women from gossiping," *The Vintage News* (blog), May 5, 2016, https://www.thevintagenews.com/2016/05/05/scolds-bridle-the-gruesome-medieval-torture-instrument-worn-to-deter-women-from-gossiping/.

48 "The Heretic's Fork," *Torture Museum* (blog), accessed October 17, 2017, http://torturemuseum.net/en/the-heretics-fork/.

they are period pieces that are often replaced with gags. Gags can be used to restrict the speech of loquacious slaves, humiliate them through loss of control over drooling, or cause them pain by holding their jaws open for a long period of time. Primarily, however, they are used for sensory deprivation rather than torture, and will be covered more extensively in Chapter 10.

## TUTORIALS

### 1. Device Bondage Hogtie

1.1 Secure wrist and ankle cuffs on your partner.

1.2 Attach wrist cuffs together with a double-ended snap hook.

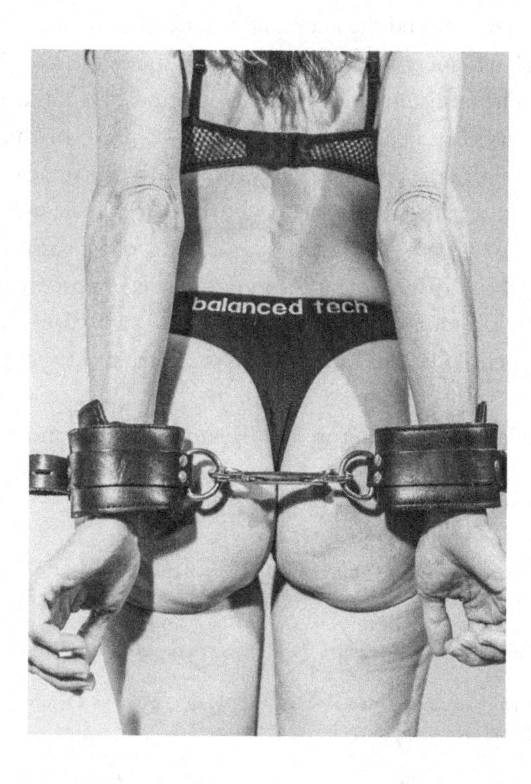

1.3 Attach ankle cuffs together with a double-ended snap hook.

1.4 Have your partner lie down comfortably on a bed, or some pillows. Attach their ankles to their wrists using carabiners. If you want to restrict their movement more, use fewer carabiners to give them less slack.

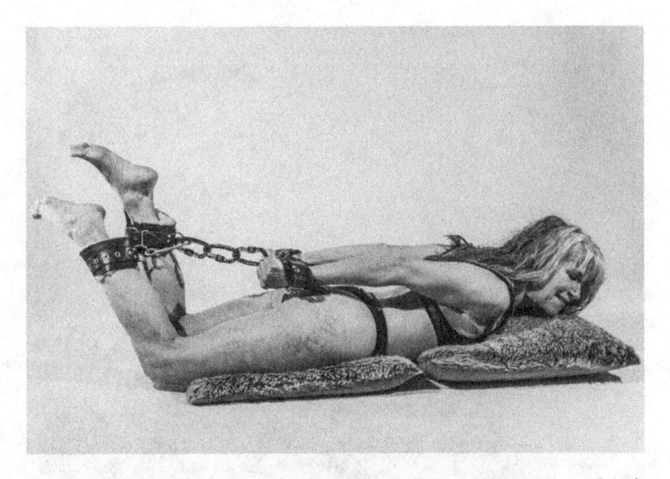

*Bottom: Simone. Top: Mistress Couple*

**Safety precautions:** Holding this position is strenuous. Make sure that you check in frequently with your partner about their circulation and breathing.

## 2. Crotch Rope

2.1 Make a bight in the rope by folding the rope in half.

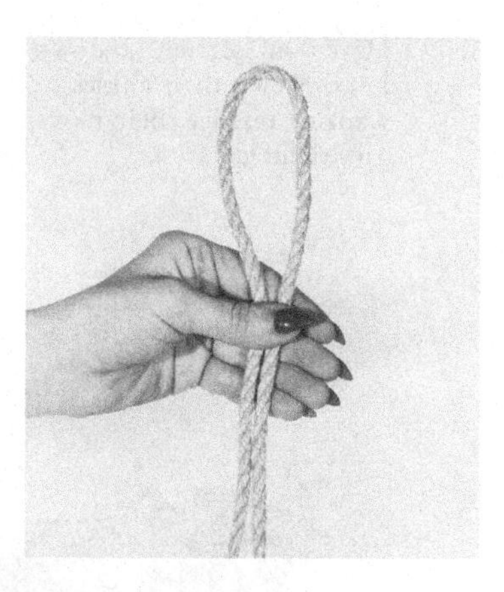

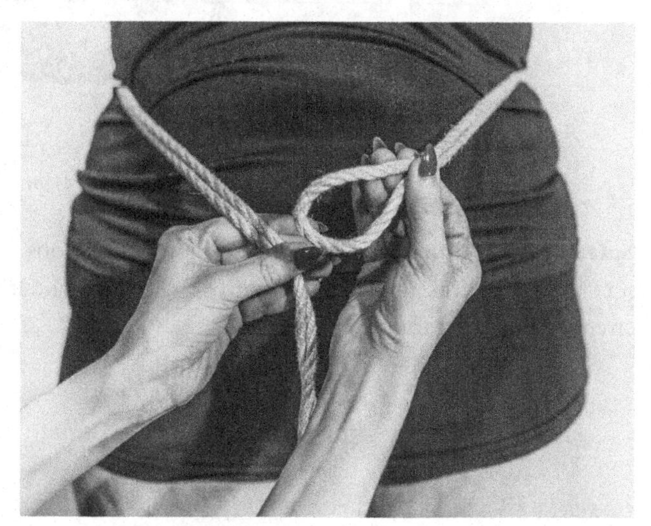

2.2 Find your bottom's waist and place the rope on it. The rope should sit right in the notch of the waist.

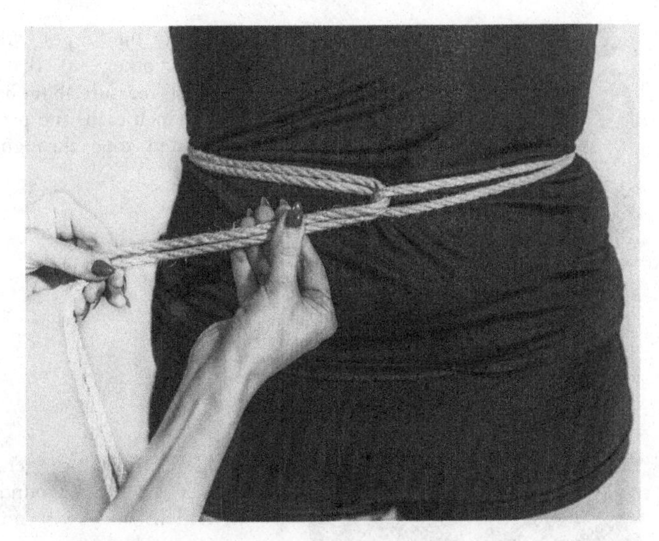

2.3 Pass the running ends of the rope through the bight and reverse the tension by pulling the rope back in the direction it just came from. This will tighten and cinch the rope.

2.4 Using the running ends, make a U shape that passes behind the rope at the waist that you want to lock onto.

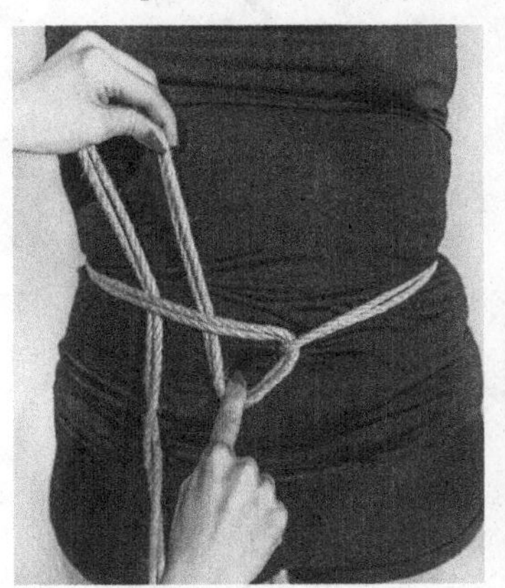

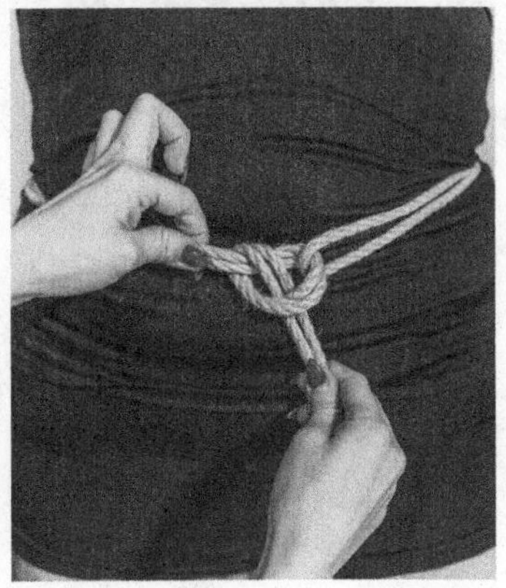

2.5 Pass the running ends over the rope that you're locking onto, and through the U shape to secure a lark's head knot.

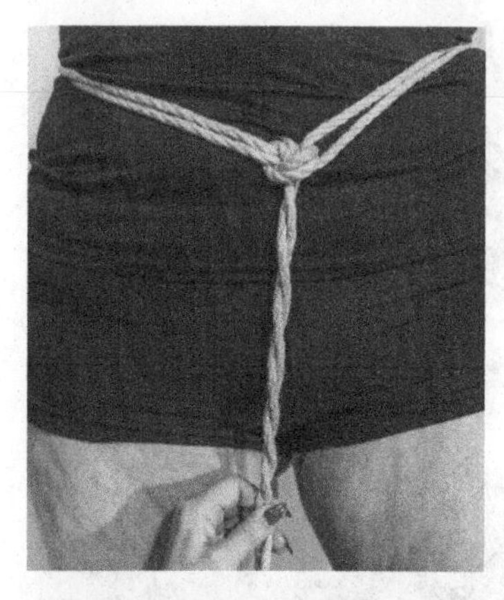

2.6 Twist the ropes around each other, so that the twists measure about half to one inch each, and pass the twisted rope through the legs.

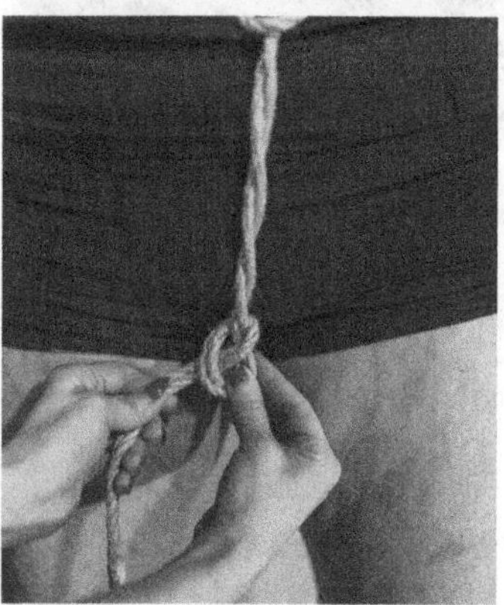

2.7 For protruding genitals: split the ropes around the genitals and twist on the other side to secure around the bulge. For nonprotruding genitals: Tie some appropriately placed overhand knots in the rope for added stimulation, and continue twisting.

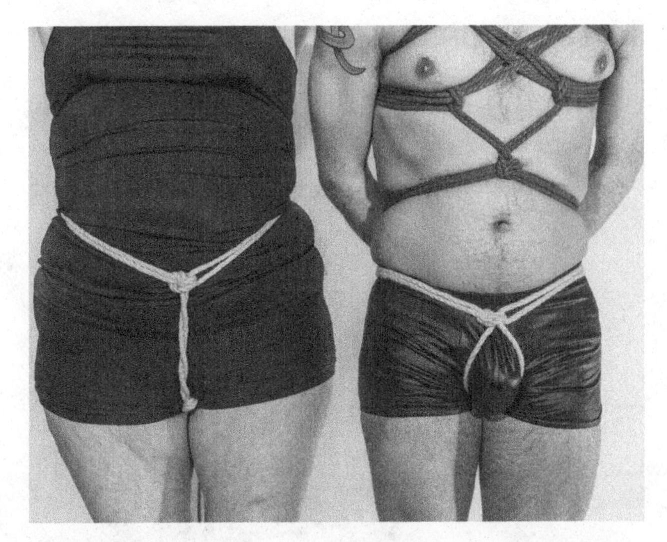

2.8 Bring the rope up through your partner's butt crack (yes, it will feel like a wedgie!), and tie another lark's head knot to secure.

*Bottoms: Rocky and Hum. Top: Mistress Couple*

**Safety precautions:** This isn't a particularly dangerous tie, but it does restrict bathroom use, so make sure that your partner uses the bathroom before tying them like this!

## 3. Toothpick Heretic's Fork

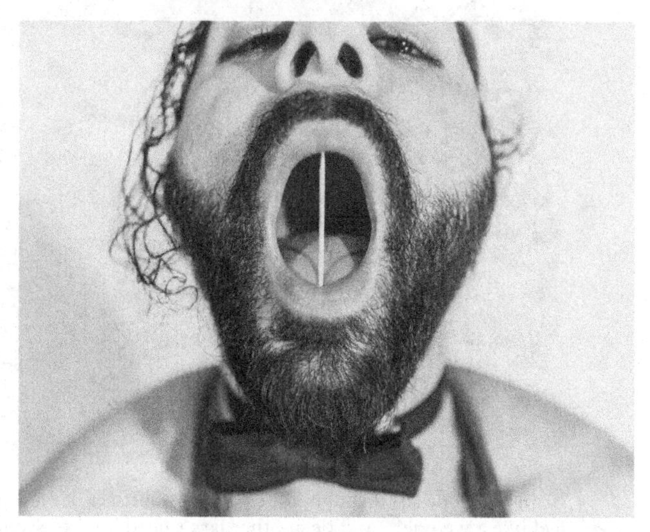

*Bottom: Hum. Top: Mistress Couple*

3.1 Have your partner open their mouth as wide as possible. Adjust toothpick for height depending on their mouth size. If they have a small mouth, you might have to break the toothpick so that it is smaller. Make sure there are no splinters sticking out if you do this.

3.2 Place the toothpick inside your partner's mouth between the top hard palate and bottom soft palate. They will have to either hold their mouth open as wide as possible to avoid pain, or accept the fact that the toothpick will be poking them.

3.3 As your partner's mouth gets tired, gravity will force it to bear down onto the toothpick, causing a great deal of pain. A smart bottom will figure out that all they have to do to relieve the pressure is to knock it out with their tongue, but for some reason people are usually so stunned by the sensation that this obvious solution completely evades them!

**Safety precautions:** I have never left someone with a toothpick in their mouth for more than five minutes and do not advise that you do so.

CHAPTER

5

# MENTAL BONDAGE

Mental bondage is one of the activities that put the *D* for discipline in BDSM. It could also be said that it represents two other D words—devotion and dominance. This is because, unlike rope bondage or device bondage, mental bondage is not physically imposed. Rather, it requires that the submissive act based on the will of the Dominant partner. Motivators for the submissive's behavior can include the desire to please, fear of punishment, and loyalty to a mutual agreement.

Many people mistake mental bondage as a "safe" form of bondage because there are no tools involved that could maim or physically injure someone, but that is far from the truth. Because mental bondage deals with a deep mental connection between Top and bottom, the possibility exists that either partner can be mentally or emotionally damaged. Sometimes these hurts can last longer and affect someone's daily routine more than physical injuries. Therefore, it is imperative that those engaging in mental bondage do so ethically, and with great care for their partners' emotional well-being. It is also very important to realize that mental bondage is a separate beast from abusive behavior, or what is referred to as psychological bondage. Whereas psychological bondage is nonconsensual, and is perpetuated through feelings of self-doubt, self-loathing, and unworthiness, consensual mental bondage can be used as an antidote to those feelings. By using the devotion to the Dominant partner as a motivator, submissive individuals can be assigned training tasks that contribute to their confidence building and add to their self-worth.

In this chapter, you will learn about contracts, position training, and hypnosis, all of which are examples of mental bondage. Due to the extensive nature of producing a contract or learning hypnosis, tutorials on those topics will not be provided.

## Contracts

BDSM relationship contracts and training regimens are very good examples of mental bondage. In fact, contracts are common social tools that have an element of bondage lurking beneath the seemingly prosaic surface. A contract, by definition, is a voluntary agreement that is enforceable (sometimes by law) as a binding accord. The use of the word *binding* to describe contracts demonstrates the inherent involvement of bondage in the concept. Whereas contracts for many types of relationship agreements are legally upheld, consensual slavery is not legally viewed as a relationship and is not considered to be legally binding anywhere in the United States.[49] Therefore, the purpose of entering into a BDSM relationship contract is not to legally entrap someone, but rather to help guide the relationship. It enables both partners to express clearly what they'd like from the arrangement and what they expect from each other. The document holds moral authority within the relationship but requires

49 "Are BDSM Contracts Legally Binding?," BDSM Contracts. 2013. Accessed October 20, 2017. https://bdsmcontracts.org/are-bdsm-contracts-legally-binding/.

devotion and active participation by both partners in order to be effective. If a partner is not willing to uphold the arrangement, it becomes null. Even if the Dominant overreaches their power by including a termination clause that prohibits a slave from terminating/canceling, the slave can still walk away at any time. Despite this legal reality, relationship contracts are wonderful examples of how bondage can be implemented without the use of physical restraint. The brain is the control center for the rest of the body, so why not just cut to the chase and control the brain?

## Position Training

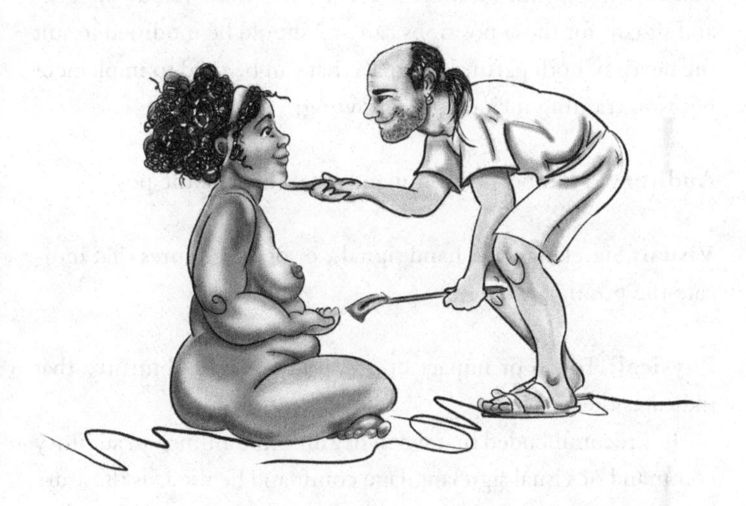

Another area of mental bondage that plays into power exchange relationships is position training, or teaching your partner a number of poses that you find to be visually appealing or useful. This type of activity is most commonly implemented in Master/slave (M/s) relationships, wherein it is referred to as "slave position training," but it can also be used in more casual dynamics. Although many older players in the BDSM community use

Gorean slave positions from John Norman's *Gor* book series as a default, there is no one right way to approach position training. Just as in any training dynamic, it is up to the Top to find rules and restrictions that suit their needs and then train their bottom to use them. Each position should have a stated purpose, as well as a punishment associated with failing to perform it properly and a reward for success. This punishment/reward system is the element that motivates the bottom to honor their commitment, and should not be overlooked.

A wonderful result of the customizable structure of position training is that it is accessible to a variety of body types that other bondage might not be suitable for. Positions as well as the cues and signals for those positions can and should be modified to suit the needs of both partners. Signals that can be used to implement position training include the following:

**Auditory:** Numbers or commands that indicate the position

**Visual:** Sign language, hand signals, or other gestures that indicate the position

**Physical:** Touch or impact on the body of the submissive that indicates the position

It is recommended that when beginning training, an auditory command or visual sign language command be used, as those are the simplest to recognize and memorize. As the bottom becomes accustomed to the training regimen, associating numbers or physical cues can be a fun way to ramp up the difficulty.

For more information about communication systems and how to use them, please refer to Chapter 2.

***Types of Training Positions:***

**Instruction:** Instruction positions are used specifically for training and communicating subjects of importance. The most commonly recognized instruction position is the military "attention." Other forms of the position, such as a "teach" position that involves taking out a notebook and writing implement, are also acceptable. Either way, when the command is given for instruction positions, it is a signal to the bottom to focus on the Top's commands or instructions intently.

**Parking:** Parking positions are to be assumed when a bottom is not carrying out an order or actively serving the Top. When parked, the bottom simply awaits the next command. It can become tedious for the Top to have to park the bottom after each and every order. Consequently, many Tops train the bottom to automatically park after completing a task.

**Mindfulness:** Mindfulness positions are very specific physical representations of the desired headspace for the submissive—for instance, keeping one's chin up to denote self-confidence, or bowing the head to demonstrate humility. Mindfulness positions are best implemented as parking positions that the bottom can start a scene with or default to when they don't know what else to do. This way, they are constantly engaged in the mental bondage rather than slouching or standing around untethered. By taking the bottom out of their everyday modes of gesture and physical expression, the Top may guide them into subspace more easily. This process of starting and parking in the position also helps the bottom to stay in the headspace that the Top desires for them throughout the scene.

**Objectification:** Objectification positions are also referred to as "inspection" or "examination" positions. They are implemented in order to take away the bottom's sense of bodily autonomy by making not only their skin, but their mouth, ears, feet, genitals, and anal area accessible to the Top. Objectification positions can be used to ensure proper hygiene, check grooming instructions, examine marks and bruises from play, or simply emotionally charge the bottom. Depending on the person, being objectified can produce intense emotions such as lust, pride, embarrassment, or humiliation. Just make sure that your partner has consented to being emotionally charged in these ways before objectifying them. Objectification positions can also be used to "transform" bottoms into human furniture ("table" or "footrest"), or reinforce animal role play ("sit, Fido!"). It is important to note that bottoms have varied reactions to objectification, anywhere along the spectrum from being deeply disturbed to wildly turned on, so Tops should make sure to check in about it during negotiation before implementing this kind of position.

**Play-oriented:** Play-oriented positions are shortcuts for the positions that the bottom will find themselves in during play. By implementing these types of positions, the Top can keep play streamlined by avoiding long-winded explanations of how they want the bottom positioned. Examples of play-oriented positions include "wrists" for presenting the wrists in imaginary shackles, "cross" for spreading oneself as if on a St. Andrew's cross, "kneel" for changing levels, and "spank" for presenting the buttocks. These positions can also be implemented with dungeon furniture and toys as a way to align the bottom before adding physically imposed bondage.

**Punishment:** Punishment positions are used for behavioral modification. Often physically stressful, these positions can become more painful over time. By altering the duration of the position, the punishment can be customized to fit the severity of the indiscretion. In some cases, punishment positions are not physically stressful but are an indication of pain/punishment (such as a spanking) that is about to come. Because many bottoms enjoy spanking, it is important to differentiate actual punishment from "funishment" or role-play punishment. The implementation of a punishment posture in conjunction with an activity that the bottom finds to be displeasurable is the best way to make this distinction.

## Erotic Hypnosis

Another wonderfully accessible form of mental bondage is erotic hypnosis. Unlike other types of mental bondage, physical states and sensations can be induced in the bottom through erotic hypnosis. For this reason, erotic hypnosis is a powerful tool for fulfilling fantasies that are too dangerous or are impeded by physical limitations.

It's important to note that erotic hypnosis is viewed as recreational rather than therapeutic. However, it does carry many of the same principles as the latter. Theories explaining what occurs during hypnosis fall into two groups. "Altered state" theories see hypnosis as an altered state of mind, or trance, whereas the more skeptical "nonstate" theories see hypnosis as a form of imaginative role play.[50] Despite the fact that "altered state" theories are viewed with more authority within the hypnosis community and "nonstate" theories are usually ascribed to by disbelievers, both have similar goals to BDSM play, and both can be experienced as erotic. Because my personal beliefs align more with the "altered state" theory, for the purposes of this book, discussion of hypnosis is going to proceed based on that paradigm.

So, what is erotic hypnosis? Hypnosis is usually applied by a procedure known as hypnotic induction, involving a series of

---

50 Steven J. Lynn and Judith W. Rhue, eds., *Theories of Hypnosis: Current Models and Perspectives* (New York: The Guilford Press, 1991).

preliminary instructions and suggestions given by the hypnotist to the subject. Once hypnotized, the subject is said to have heightened focus and concentration, as well as an increased response to suggestion from the hypnotist. It is widely accepted by "altered state" theorists that this mental state is a form of trance. Interestingly, studies have shown that arousal is also a type of trance.[51] As you know, there are many ways to become aroused, or to reach an arousal trance. Some people prefer to become aroused through direct physical and visual stimulation, such as masturbation, kissing/petting with a partner, or watching porn. But others use shortcuts that do not involve physical contact, such as discussing eroticism with others. And more intellectualized approaches to inducing the arousal trance might employ strategies like guided visualization. These are the components of erotic hypnosis.

Erotic hypnotic suggestions are customized by the hypnotist and their subject based on their intention for play. The hypnotic language that is used can elicit sensory memories, such as the feeling of being kissed, caressed, or even bound. Recalling these memories while in trance can produce physical sensations in the body, so a hypnotized person can experience all the sensations and sexual pleasure that they would enjoy if they were actually being physically manipulated. Many hypnosubjects compare this feeling of mental and physical control with subspace. In a typical D/s subspace, emotional connection is generated through active participation. Hypnosis can amplify these feelings because the submissive can maintain a passive role but will still be able to feel the intention of the Dominant partner controlling their movements or thoughts. Whereas in typical D/s subspace, obedience is a skill that is learned and acted upon by the bottom, in

---

51 Northwestern University. "Getting into the flow: Sexual pleasure is a kind of trance: Orgasm is all about rhythmic timing." *ScienceDaily*, November 1, 2016, www.sciencedaily.com/releases/2016/11/161101103448.htm.

hypnospace, that obedience is enforced by mental bondage. The intensity of this mental bondage is known to create a deep bond between practitioners. Hypnosis bottoms often report feelings of possession by the hypnotist, and many of them elaborate that this deepens their feelings of submission toward the hypnotist.[52]

Due to the fact that erotic hypnosis is associated with passivity, many people worry about whether or not it is consensual. The thing is that, in order to be hypnotized, the bottom has to be a willing participant. In order to be a willing participant, one must have a conscious connection that allows them to understand the hypnotist's suggestions and use their imagination to enhance those suggestions, as well as an emotional connection that allows them to trust that the experience will work and that the hypnotist won't hurt them. If one of these criteria is not met, the bottom will not go into trance.[53] There are some exceptions to this, but only with very vulnerable bottoms and highly skilled or unethical Tops. Most hypnotized people remember everything that happens during a hypnosis session, so it is unlikely that they can be taken advantage of while in the trance. Many people also have the ability to recognize danger and get out of harm's way while in the trance, and have even been reported to avoid people they dislike.[54] While these abilities might confuse onlookers into thinking that hypnosis is fake, what they suggest is that the hypnotized person is conscious and connected to himself or herself.

Overall, hypnosis is an advanced practice that requires hours

---

52 Daniel, "Erotic Hypnosis—What It Is, and Why You Should You [sic] Try It," *Hypnotic Dreams* (blog), November 10, 2017, https://www.hypnoticdreams.com/erotic-hypnosis/.

53 Nathalie Rupert, "Hypnosis and Consent: It's All About What You Believe," National Coalition for Sexual Freedom (blog), February 25, 2017, http://www.ncsfreedom.org/press/blog/item/guest-blog-hypnosis-and-consent-it-s-all-about-what-you-believe.

54 Ibid.

of study to achieve mastery. Because of this, I won't be going into instructions on how to do it. If you want to pursue erotic hypnosis, make sure that you learn basic hypnosis techniques from a qualified instructor, and that you practice nonerotic hypnosis with your partner first to build trust and confidence.

Hypnosis is one of the many fetishes that experienced a boom in the early 2000s as the internet and AOL chat rooms created venues for closeted individuals to share their interests.[55] Because of this, the internet has been flooded with millions of hypnosis scripts that other hypnosis practitioners have used and achieved success with. Most practitioners recommend that beginner and even intermediate level practitioners use a script so that they can focus on the subject rather than what they're going to say next. Another benefit of using hypnosis scripts is that they have advanced hypnotic techniques such as induction, relaxation deepening, programming exercises (to accomplish the goals set for the session), exit processes, and posthypnotic suggestion to extend the benefits of the session directly built into the text.[56] Using scripts will help you get acquainted with different hypnosis techniques before you're comfortable with improvising. As in any BDSM activity, always stick to prenegotiated agreements, and potentially even build those agreements into your script.

---

55 Ibid.

56 Mandy Bass, "Self Hypnosis Script to Get the Most Out of Your Practice," *Mind to Succeed* (blog), accessed November 20, 2017, https://www.mindtosucceed.com/self-hypnosis-script.html.

Suggested areas of exploration of erotic hypnosis include the following:

**Sexual enhancement:** Hypnotic suggestions can include techniques to reduce inhibitions, increase arousal, or even trigger physical responses such as orgasm. Many D/s couples who are interested in orgasm control or orgasm on command use erotic hypnosis as a tool in that quest.

**Fantasy fulfillment:** Subjects can be placed in a trance and taken through the description of a sexual experience to the point where they physically experience it. Depending on the willingness of the bottom and the skill level of the Top, such an experience might be as realistic as feeling bound and restrained, or as fantastical as being suspended in a spiderweb and devoured by the black widow herself.

**Personality transformation:** Hypnotic suggestions help the subject to imagine themselves as someone else and assume a different personality or identity. While role play is one way to achieve this escape from self, hypnosis enhances the experience by helping the subject get into character and stay in it. This makes the scene feel more realistic. Most transformations only last the length of a scene, but some people, like those who are exploring gender roles, can use erotic hypnosis to effect more permanent changes like variations in tone of voice or shedding layers of gendered conditioning.

## TUTORIALS

### 1. Position Training

Teach your bottom a variety of training positions that work for their body. Have them practice transitioning from one position to the next as gracefully as possible.

Balance a ring on their head, collar, or shoulder, and see if they can perform the same transitions without dropping the ring. If they cannot, see if they can perform the same transitions without dropping the ring more than a certain number of times. Have them practice until they are able to perform the transitions with consistency.

Once you are satisfied that they are consistently performing the transitions without dropping the ring, ascribe power to the ring by declaring a punishment for dropping it. The punishment must be proportional to the task that you're asking the bottom to perform and their ability to do it.

For instance, if your partner usually drops the ring up to five times within a transition period, threatening no orgasms for a week if they drop the ring once is too harsh a punishment and will discourage them from participating. A more appropriate punishment would be no orgasms for the rest of the night or some sort of pain infliction if they drop the ring more than five times.

Adjust the punishment system based on skill level and increase the level of difficulty as needed.

## 2. Mantra Training, a Precursor to Hypnosis

Fill in the blanks:

The purpose of a (bottom's title) is to (action) and to (action) for (Top's title) for (duration of time).

**Examples:**

The purpose of a slave is to be as hot as Mistress wants and to serve Mistress's pleasures at all times.

The purpose of a puppy is to be obedient and protect Master while collared.

The purpose of a painslut is to be open and available for Mistrix to use whenever they please.

The purpose of a sissy maid is to clean and tidy for Sir on Tuesdays and Saturdays.

The purpose of a newbie is to clearly report what I am experiencing to my Top at all times.

Have the bottom sit in a predetermined posture and repeat the mantra over and over again (out loud or silently) until they are in a relaxed state. Reciting a mantra is a powerful mind-training tool that will remind the bottom of what to focus on during the bondage experiment. While this exercise only skims the surface of the mental control that one can achieve through hypnosis, it does train the mind to focus and can add a sexy mental bondage aspect to any scene.

CHAPTER

6

# OBJECTIFICATION BONDAGE

The concept of sexual objectification and, in particular, the objectification of women is a hot topic of discussion in today's society. Many feminists regard sexual objectification as deplorable and as playing an important role in gender inequality. In fact, the fight against the sexual objectification of women has become one of the most prominent social issues in the United States since the 2016 election. However, some social commentators argue that modern women objectify themselves as an expression of their empowerment, and therefore such objectification should be considered feminist. The key element that explains these differing viewpoints is that of consent.

There's a distinct difference between unknowingly being reduced to a sexual object and consensually engaging in the decision to participate in such an activity. Often, nonconsensual sexual objectification is perpetrated by individuals who view the subject primarily as an object of their desire rather than a whole person. This type of treatment can often lead to negative psychological effects, including eating disorders, depression, and sexual dysfunction. Victims of nonconsensual sexual objectification usually experience a diminishing of self-worth due to the belief that their intelligence and competence are not being acknowledged by society. By choosing to engage in sexual objectification, the subject reverses these effects. They are able to exhibit bodily autonomy and personal agency by choosing how they want to be objectified and by whom. The power involved in making such decisions with a partner who does see the entirety of one's personhood can be incredibly healing and enriching.

People of color, transgender people, and women are the most common victims of nonconsensual sexual objectification, and therefore arguably stand to gain the most from consensual sexual objectification if they choose to do so. This does not exclude white cisgender males from the population that benefits from consensual sexual objectification. In fact, degradation and objectification are often the sexual activities of choice among many high-powered white businessmen because they are wonderful tools for disengaging from an active mind and integrating into the body.

We will begin our exploration into objectification bondage through the lens of Aristotle, one of the most noted and respected white men to (allegedly) benefit from the activity in the form of animal role play. Then we will explore what animal role play and the equally objectifying furniture role-play activities entail, and learn about some fun ways to incorporate them into BDSM play. Finally, we will discuss bondage positions that are intended specifically for sexual objectification and romps in the bedroom. Something to keep in mind as you read is that most of the bondage activities that we have read about so far focus on restraint. While objectification bondage contains elements of restraint, it also focuses heavily on adornment and the headspace that being decorated or transformed can have on the psyche. Learning about objectification bondage will serve as a useful bridge to costume bondage and other forms of bondage that focus less on restraint.

## "The Aristotelian Perversion"

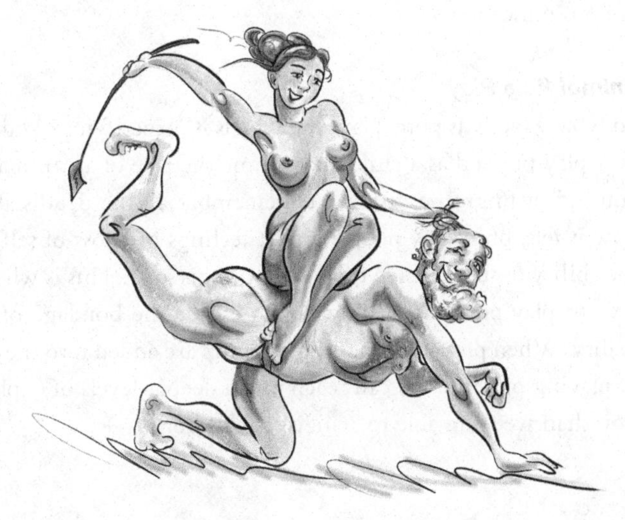

According to legend, Aristotle was tutoring young Alexander the Great when he scolded Alexander for paying more attention to his mistress than to his studies. Upon hearing that he had made these comments, the beautiful young mistress, Phyllis, vowed to exact her revenge on Aristotle for intervening in her relationship. One day, she sneaked into Aristotle's study and seduced the old philosopher into letting her ride him like a horse. Some versions of the legend include an ending wherein, at Phyllis's insistence, Alexander hid and secretly watched his mentor's humiliation at her hand.[57] Other versions, especially artistic depictions of the legend, reference Aristotle's joy in the role reversal from powerful philosopher to the objectified pet of a beautiful woman. In fact, this image became a very popular trope in classical art and can be found depicted in a variety of mediums throughout the ages. Thus, pony play became known

57 "Aristotle Ridden by Phyllis," Feminae: Medieval Women and Gender Index, accessed October 19, 2017, https://inpress.lib.uiowa.edu/feminae/DetailsPage.aspx?Feminae_ID=32244.

as the "Aristotelian perversion" due to its association with the famous philosopher.

### *Animal Role Play*

So what exactly is pony play, and why is it objectifying? Did you ever play pretend as a child and assume the role of an animal? If you did, it might be difficult to remember all the details about how it felt, but many people report feelings of a loss of self and the ability to step outside their everyday persona. This is why we love to play pretend: It allows us to escape the bondage of our reality. When power-exchange dynamics are added into the mix of playing pretend, we can reach much deeper levels of exploration than we were able to achieve as children.

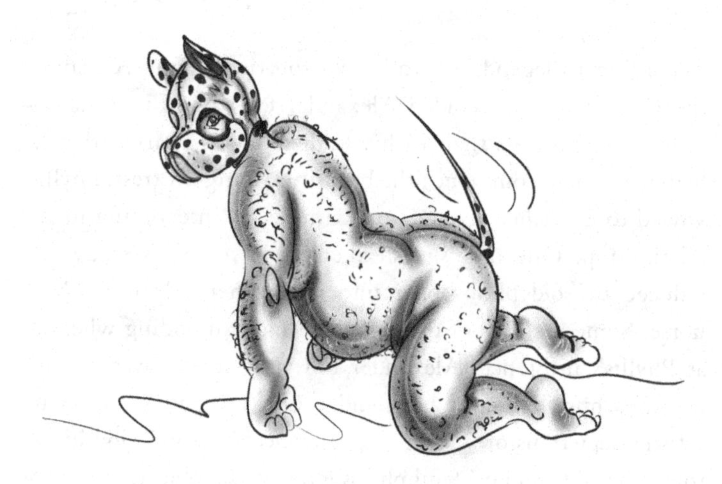

Playing the role of an owned animal can be incredibly objectifying. Doing so strips one of their human identity and turns them into a pet for their owner to use and admire. Therefore, this type of animal role play is often referred to as pet play. Pet play is seen as separate from other nonobjectifying forms of animal role play such as primal play and furry play. Yes, you read that correctly. Not all forms of animal role play are objectifying. In fact, the reasons for playing an animal can vary quite a bit. As previously stated, some people enjoy being able to cut loose into a more dynamic personality, while for others there is a spiritual element to it. Some enjoy the masochistic exercise of enduring the labor of a farm animal, while others seek to be stroked, rubbed, and held like an adored lap pet. It is also important to note that not all animal role players assume a submissive or bottoming role—think Catwoman or Wolverine. All this being said, a lot of what determines the levels of objectification within the play scenario, besides the attitudes of the players, is the bondage equipment that is (or is not) used to transform the human into an animal.

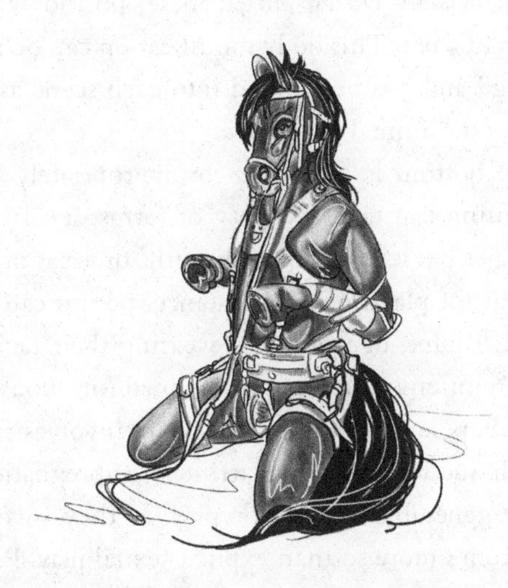

Pony play in particular utilizes a lot of bondage equipment. Whether the participants identity as workhorses, riding horses, or show horses, different types of modified horse tack including bridles, bit gags, saddles, and reins can all be used to help train them. Bit gags are incredibly objectifying, as they strip you of your ability to control salivation and cause you to drool like an animal. Some human ponies find drooling on themselves to be humiliating, while others find it to be quite erotic.

Other popular species involved in pet play include canines (puppies, dogs, wolves), felines (kittens, big cats), and bovines (cows, bulls), but the options are limitless. One of my favorite pet-play bondage scenarios of all time involved a human pet seal trying to balance a ball on his nose while slapping his tail (legs bound together) on the ground. Now that's a predicament! That scene was a wonderful example of bondage-based body modification that was utilized to objectify the participant. Other forms of bondage-based body modification that can be used in a similar way are prosthetic hooves or mitts to strip the human of the privilege of opposable thumbs, tail-shaped plugs, or the tying of limbs in a *futomomo* ("fat leg" in Japanese) position to resemble the short legs of a pet. This body modification can be referred to as "grooming" and can be worked into each scene as a gradual warm-up into the animal headspace.

Once the bottom is tacked up or appropriately bound for play, pet training can take a variety of forms. That being said, each type of pet has its particular strengths or areas of focus that can steer ideas for playtime. For instance, ponies can be taught how to walk, canter, or trot while wearing their tack. Puppies and kittens are often trained and disciplined (or "housebroken") by their handlers, and bovine play usually involves fantasies of milking with suction cups and artificial impregnation. These activities are generally seen as foreplay, as they involve subtle erotic undertones more so than explicit sexual play. Pet play has nothing to do with bestiality or sexual attraction to animals, and thus sex play is often reserved for the closing grooming activity, after the subject has been unbound and returned to their human physical form.

## Furniture Role Play

Forniphilic creations (or human furniture) have been referenced in pop culture time and time again. Rewatch Marilyn Monroe's famous "Diamonds Are a Girl's Best Friend" number from *Gentlemen Prefer Blondes*, and you'll notice that the chandeliers are actually made of bound women! Salvador Dalí was once photographed sitting at a desk made from a woman in a backbend, with a pair of legs sprouting out of a potted plant behind him. The castle staff in Disney's *Beauty and the Beast* were transformed into singing and dancing furniture under the sorceress's spell. To quote that film, the forniphilia trope is a "tale as old as time."

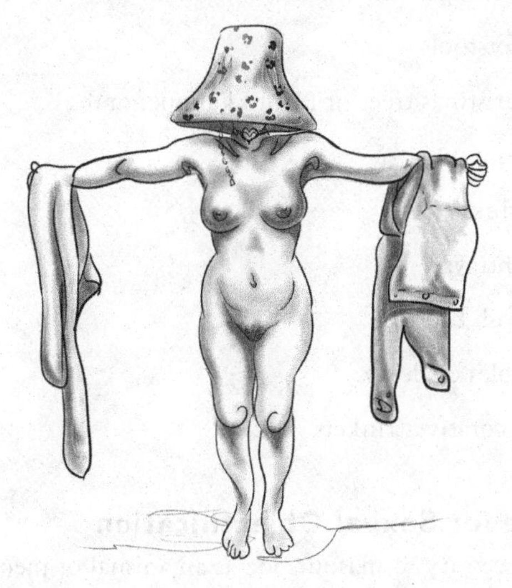

Transforming someone into human furniture puts the human form on display in an incredibly objectifying way. Whereas animal role play still allows for some personal agency over behaviors, furniture items are inanimate objects, and thus this type of role play is far more restrictive. Forniphilia is an extreme form of bondage because the subject is usually tightly bound and expected to stay immobile for a prolonged period of time. The use of forniphilic gags (such as feather dusters, toilet brushes, and serving trays), which help to transform the subject into the object of their Top's choosing, can also make it difficult to breathe when used for long periods of time. Therefore, it's important that human furniture always be supervised, unlike their lifeless counterparts.

Some popular types of forniphilic creations that you can try with your partners are:

- Sitting chairs or stools
- Rocking chairs
- Footstools
- Christmas trees or Hanukkah menorahs
- Lamps
- Drink trays
- Ashtrays
- Scrub brushes
- Tables or desks
- Decorative trinkets

## Bondage for Sexual Objectification

It is not necessary to masquerade as an animal or piece of furniture in order to be objectified. In fact, being sexually objectified for one's human form can be quite potent in the bedroom. Many people have fantasies about one partner being pinned up against the wall during sex, and while the position is not explicitly objectifying, it provides a good example of why movement restriction and sex make such great partners. If handled properly, the vulnerability that is created when one is restrained is a shortcut to creating deep intimacy between partners.

This section will show you a variety of positions that are perfect for sexual objectification and sexual play. In order to learn how to restrain someone in these positions, please use the column ties that you learned in Chapter 3 or the bondage devices that you learned about in Chapter 4. Generally, with sexual play the goal of the restraint is to pin the bottom in a position that they're comfortable holding for an extended period of time. Otherwise, you'll have to keep interrupting your scene in order to bind and unbind. If you have a partner who enjoys a challenge, some balancing predicaments can be added into the mix. The following positions are listed in order from least to most challenging.

- **Chair bondage:** Chair bondage is a fantastic position for beginners. Chair bondage creates a deep sense of vulnerability with the added luxury of comfort. The position can be maintained for extended periods of time, since the person is sitting. Typically the participant's wrists are tied to the arms of the chair and their ankles are tied to the legs of the chair to create a splayed-out effect, but this can be modified to suit a variety of body types and fantasies. Due to the seated position, this position can limit penetrative sexual acts. Some bondage furniture is designed to work around this and provide penetrative access, for instance by including a hole in the seat of the chair. You can also work around this by preplacing insertables before restraining your partner, or gearing the play toward other types of sexual intercourse such as oral sex or stimulation with vibrators.[58]

---

58 Stella Harris, "8 Bondage Sex Positions from Simple to Extreme!" *Kinkly* (blog), June 9, 2017, https://www.kinkly.com/8-bondage-sex-positions-from-simple-to-extreme/2/14792.

- **Spread eagle:** Thanks to the popularity of the musical *Chicago*, many people are familiar with position "number seventeen, the spread eagle!" Already viewed as a salacious sexual position, the spread eagle becomes far more objectifying when incorporating bondage. In this position, your partner can lie faceup or facedown, after which your partner's limbs are secured to the four corners of your bed (see Chapter 4 on device bondage for ideas on how best to bind your partner). Just take note that circulation can be impaired whenever your partner's arms are above their heart. Check in frequently with your partner to make sure that the restraints aren't too tight and that they aren't experiencing any coldness, numbness, or dizziness. In fact, this activity might be the perfect time to break out the fuzzy wrist and ankle cuffs.

- **Bent and spread:** In ancient Rome, sexual positions that bent at the waist were known as "coitus more ferarum" or "sexual intercourse in the manner of wild beasts."[59] Today many refer to it as "doggy style," confirming the notion that bent and spread positions bring out the beast in us. Depending on whether the partner is permitted to kneel or forced to stand, the level of difficulty in maintaining this position can be adjusted. Similarly, where the hands are placed and whether or not they offer additional support to the position can determine the level of difficulty. In order to make this sort of tie more accessible, bind someone so that they can bend at the waist and rest their torso on the bed. To increase the difficulty, use a spreader bar to keep the legs locked in a wide stance,

---

59 Robert J. Campbell, "Coitus more ferarum," Campbell's Psychiatric Dictionary (Oxford University Press, 2009), 204.

or tilt the body off balance by securing the wrists to the ankles or to the spreader bar itself. Ankle-to-wrist positions are the best for transitioning during a scene without having to unbind and rebind. If your partner is getting uncomfortable holding a certain pose, simply tip them over onto their side or back and continue the fun!

- **Gagged:** As mentioned in the animal role-play section, gags can be incredibly objectifying tools of bondage. They manipulate the mouth, the universally penetrable hole, no matter what type of body. By either filling the mouth or holding it open, gags objectify this body part as a tool for sexual pleasure and stimulation. Gags can be used on their own or worked into other types of restraint. Make sure you're using a nonverbal communication system if your partner is gagged, and look out for teeth and jaw issues. Luckily, gags come in a variety of materials as well as styles, so you can choose one that is equally comfortable and objectifying to suit your needs.

## TUTORIALS

### 1. Balloon Bouncy Chair

1.1 Blow up twenty to thirty folding balloons.

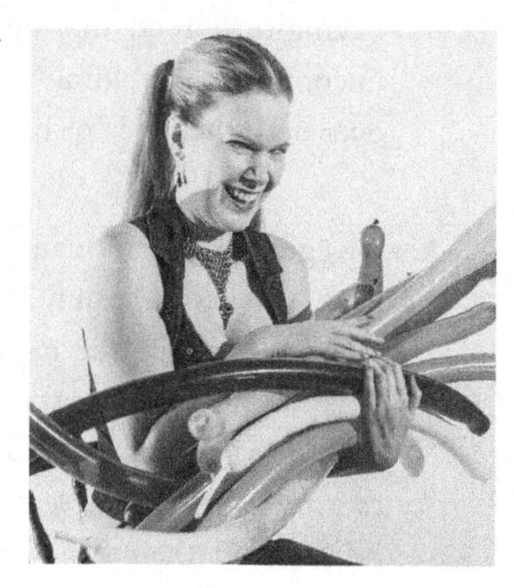

1.2 Have your bottom sit comfortably in a chair.

1.3 You can create a balloon blindfold by twisting balloons over your bottom's face. Just make sure that their eyes are closed when you're doing this.

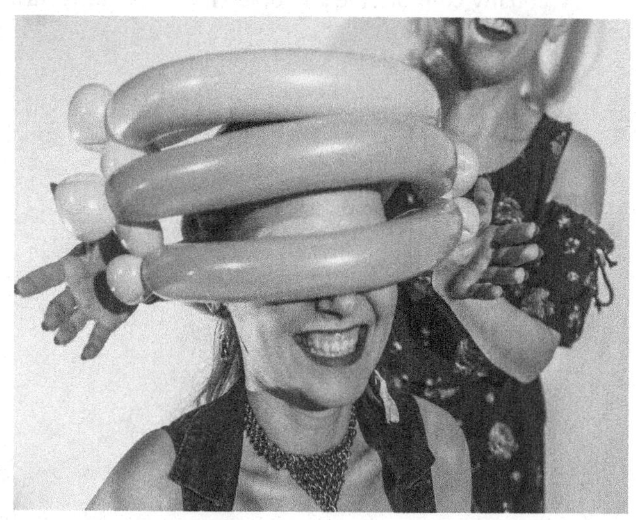

1.4 Using the single- and double-column techniques from Chapter 3, secure the bottom to the chair by twisting the balloons to lock them into place. You can be as creative as you'd like with the placement, and use as many or as few balloons as you see fit to restrain the bottom.

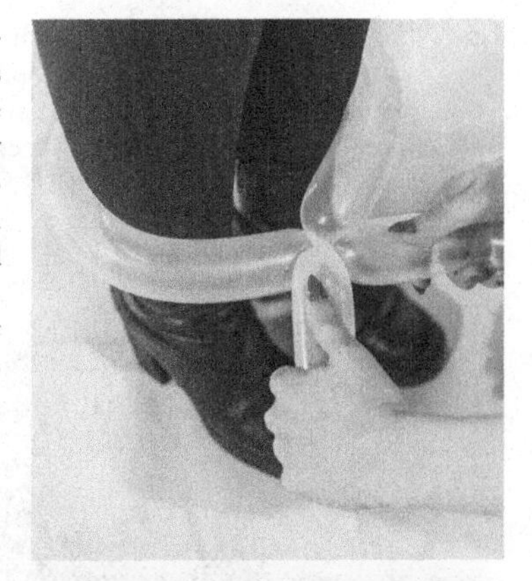

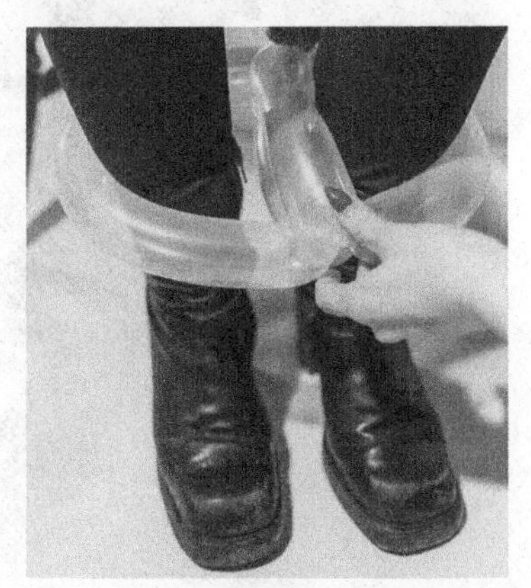

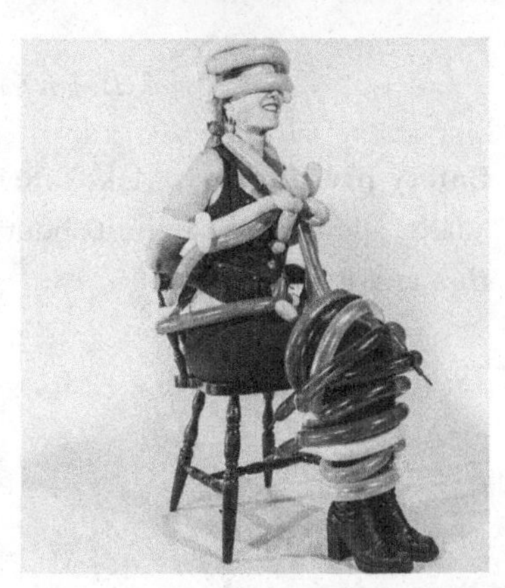

1.5 Sit on your new chair and bounce away! What a great tease! Be careful that if the balloons pop, they will tighten around the bottom like a tourniquet. This shouldn't cause any immediate damage, but you won't want to keep them on for too long.

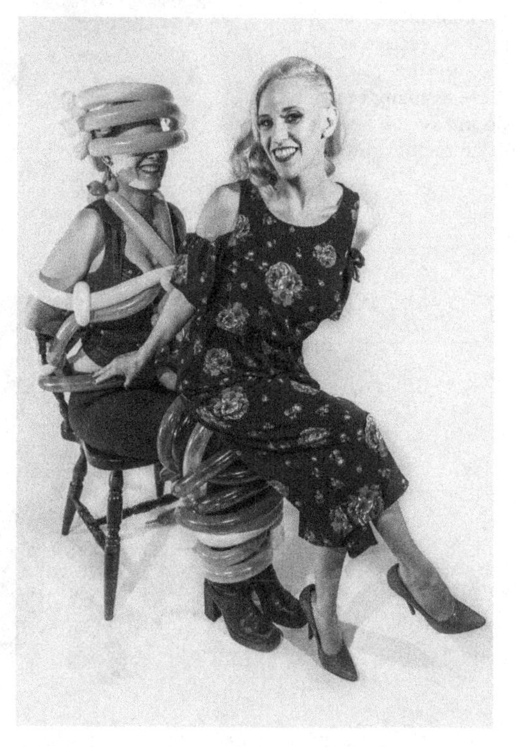

*Bottom: Duchess Jealoquin. Top: Mistress Couple*

**Safety precautions:** Make sure that your partner does not have a latex allergy or hard limit about loud noises before engaging in this activity.

## 2. Pet Play Futomomo

2.1 Have the bottom sit with their feet on the floor and their legs bent.

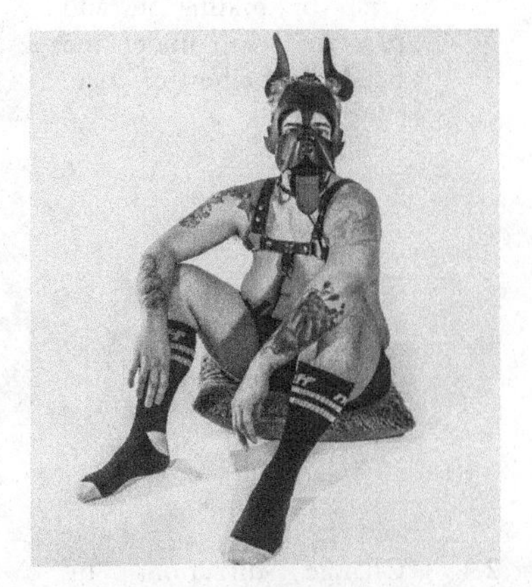

2.2 Using plastic wrap or pallet wrap, tightly wrap clockwise around the bent arm or leg.

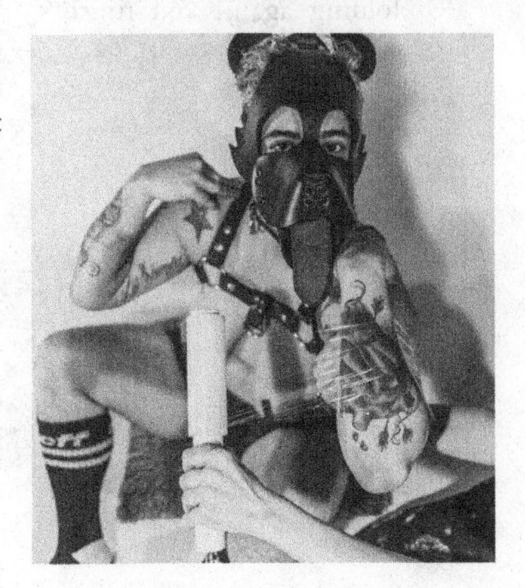

2.3 Change directions of the wrap by folding it, and pass the wrap under the bend in the elbow or knee.

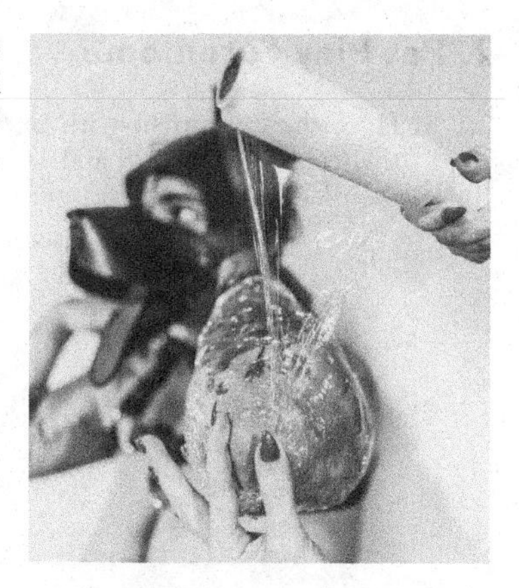

2.4 Change directions by folding again, and finish wrapping the arm or leg.

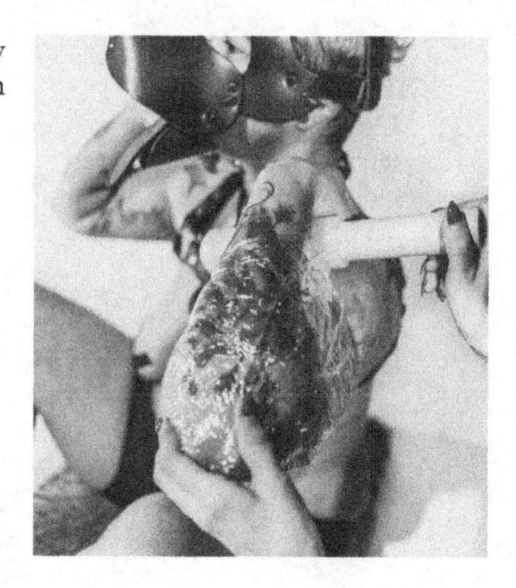

2.5 Stick wrap to itself.

2.6 Repeat the process on other limbs.

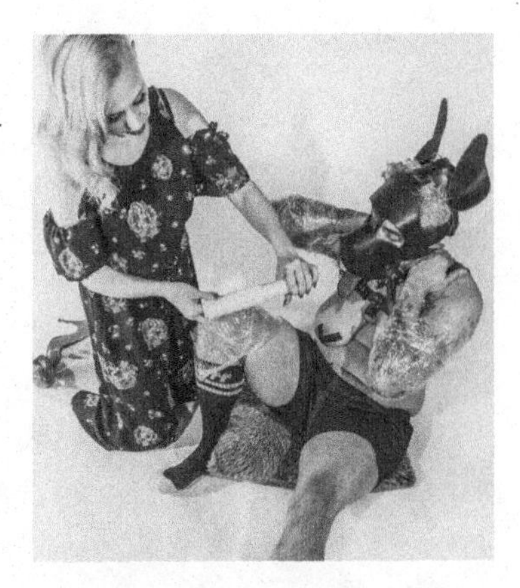

2.7 Let your pet try to locomote, play fetch, sit, roll over!

2.8 Use safety shears or unwind to remove.

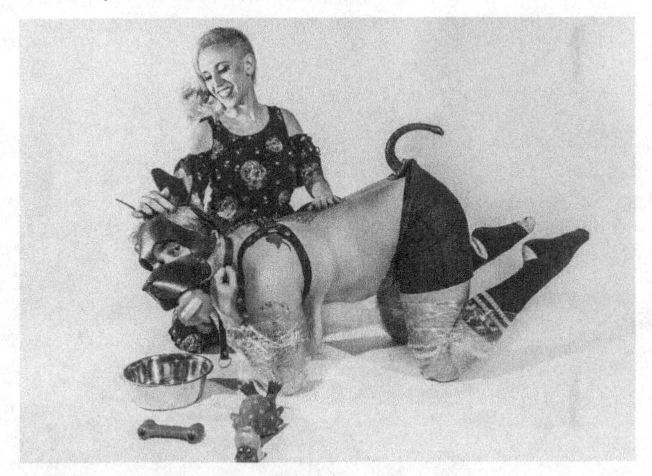

*Bottom: Gage. Top: Mistress Couple.*

**Safety precautions:** Being restrained in a bent position and bearing weight on the limbs can cause muscles or joints to feel crampy or achy if left for too long. This is meant to be a short-term activity, so check in about your partner's comfort levels frequently.

CHAPTER

7

# COSTUME BONDAGE

Imagine that you're getting ready for a sexy date. Generally, you choose your clothing based on the image that you want to portray to your partner. If you want to send a message that you're feeling kinky, what better way than to add some elements of bondage fashion into your outfit? It shouldn't be that difficult—in recent years, as BDSM has become more widely accepted in pop culture, bondage fashion trends have been widely adopted by the general public. As fashion historian Valerie Steele pointed out in her book *Fetish: Fashion, Sex & Power*, "Fashion trendsetters . . . are drawn to the theatricality of fetishistic eroticism, the implication that merely by wearing a particular style one becomes the kind of person to whom sexual adventures happen."[60]

Bondage isn't just a new fashion fad, though; techniques have been used as adornment or accessory by all genders around the globe for thousands of years. Unfortunately, the old adage "beauty is pain" applies here, as how costume bondage makes

---

60 Valerie Steele, *Fetish: Fashion, Sex & Power* (New York: Oxford University Press, 1996), 194.

you look and how it makes you feel are typically two very different experiences. Many types of costume bondage and body modification (such as piercing, neck ringing, corsetry, and foot binding) have been used to denote social status and reflect cultural interpretations of beauty. Sadly, the same modifications that are used to enhance someone's appearance usually restrict their mobility, revealing a darker motivation behind the aesthetic preference. For instance, small waists and tiny feet, the results of tight lacing with corsets and foot binding, were seen as symbols of wealth and class because the people who engaged in them were physically immobilized to the point where they were unable to do any labor. Instead, they were objectified as desirable household items, their sole purpose reduced to be visually appealing to those around them. Physical mobility, however, was not the only thing affected by body modification. Social mobility was often controlled and prevented by specific brandings or piercings meant to denote slavery. Even today, people who consensually pierce, brand, or tattoo their own bodies might be prevented from acquiring certain jobs due to social prejudice against such modifications.

This chapter will aim to focus primarily on the decorative function of costume bondage as well how the form of each costume garment imposes bondage on the wearer. To begin with, we will discuss the history of one of the most normalized forms of bondage that exists on the planet: the wedding ring.

## Bound by Love

Arguably the most common and socially accepted form of costume bondage is the wedding ring, a symbol of union that has been used for thousands of years. Evidence suggests that early handfasting rituals and wedding ceremonies coincided with the establishment of societies around 7000 BCE. Although ancient weddings were more economic and political in nature as opposed to the modern-day emphasis on love and commitment between spouses, they were an integral type of social contract that held the growing community together. As contracts are typically referred to as "binding agreements," they can be considered one of the purest forms of psychological bondage. The application of such agreements was made through the adornment of handfasting, the predecessor of the modern wedding ring.

The term *handfasting* stems from the Old Icelandic "handfesta" or the shaking of hands to signify a contract.[61] The custom derives from the act of tying the wrists and hands of a bride and groom together during a commitment ceremony, in order to signify the social contract between them. While handfasting was originally used to commemorate a commitment ceremony or engagement rather than marriage, the ritual is likely where the modern-day euphemism "tying the knot" is derived from.

The appearance of the ring as a marital symbol did not appear until sometime later. Many jewelry manufacturers offer the romanticized claim that ancient peoples exchanged braided rings of hemp or reeds to symbolize perpetual love, though the accuracy of the claim is questionable. Ancient Greek and Roman societies are among the first proven to have used jewelry as a symbol of union.[62] This evolution in form was most certainly implemented to increase the function of the ritual object from simply a symbol of union to a form of possession. Made from precious metals, these rings were initially worn by men to symbolize power and authority, but the valuable rings were eventually used as marital dowry, or a bride price, adding the principle of property possession onto the mix.[63] According to author Charles Thompson, when the betrothal rings became associated

---

61 *Oxford English Dictionary*, s.v. "handfast," accessed May 30, 2018, http://www.oed.com/view/Entry/83839#eid1996561.

62 Barbara Jo Chesser, "Analysis of Wedding Rituals: An Attempt to Make Wedding More Meaningful," *Family Relations* 29, No. 2 (April 1980), 205.

63 Ibid.

with ownership and obedience, men stopped wearing them.[64] Though the presentation of a ring was intended to be used as a token to the pledge of fidelity from the man to the woman, the reality was quite the opposite. The function of using a heavy metal for a ring was that it would create an indent or tan line on the woman's finger, a recognizable mark, should the woman try to remove the ring for any reason. In his book, *The Hand of Destiny*, Thompson pointed out that betrothal rings were worn on the left hand. Since most people were right-hand dominant, the left hand was associated with submission and obedience.[65] Thus, the wedding ring became its own uniquely disguised form of costume bondage.

Perhaps a more romantic reason for wearing the ring on the left hand could be traced to the evidence of betrothal rings found in Egyptian tombs. Both the ancient Egyptians and Greeks were known to have performed human dissections, and in doing so, discovered a nerve running from the fourth finger on the left hand to the heart. Latin author Aulus Gellius explained that due to its connection to the heart, the fourth finger of the left hand came to be the finger that donned the betrothal ring.[66] Later, it became known as the "ring finger." Today, engagement rings are typically worn on the left hand.

Only in the twentieth century in the United States did the practice of both the wife and the husband wearing rings to symbolize a union become common practice. Following suit with form and function, the groom's ring only became a tradition in the United States "when weddings, marriage and 'masculine domesticity' became synonymous with prosperity,

---

64 Ibid.

65 Ibid.

66 Gary Vikan, "Art and Marriage in Early Byzantium," *Dumbarton Oaks Papers* Vol 44 (1990), 146.

capitalism, and national stability."[67] Today, much of the history behind wedding rings is unknown to the general public; they are viewed more as a fashion accessory than a form of bondage. However, their function remains the same as in the days of old—to bind couples to each other symbolically and practically, as their wedding vows say: "Until death do us part."

## Collars and Rings

Using rings as a form of costume bondage to denote a social contract is not a practice restricted to traditionalists. The BDSM community is known to utilize ring piercings and collars to symbolize a commitment between partners. Collars and ring piercings are often viewed as treasured items because they serve similar functions as wedding rings—property possession and objectification. By turning these functions into erotic themes to play upon, BDSM practitioners are able to reclaim the dark symbolism behind both collars and slave piercings, and breathe new meaning into them.

While those interested in participating in a long-term consensual Master/slave dynamic might adopt the practice of piercing to denote ownership, more casual play partners usually choose a less permanent form of costume bondage, such as the collar, to symbolize the commitment. Collars are made out of a variety of materials, from ribbon to the standard leather, and even heavy locking metal, so it is possible to choose one appropriate to the level of experience of the wearer. As with engagement and wedding rings, there are traditions with collars in regard to the materials and colors that are appropriate for each stage in the relationship, usually becoming more elaborate with increasing devotion.

---

67 Vicki Howard, "A Real Man's Ring: Gender and the Invention of Tradition," *Journal of Social History* 36, no. 4 (Summer 2003): 837-856, https://doi.org/10.1353/jsh.2003.0098.

Often in the BDSM community, a three-stage collaring process is used to indicate different stages in a developing relationship. Under this system, the "consideration collar" is the first collar presented to a submissive, and has no personal value attached. This is a collar that can be used by anyone. When worn, the consideration collar serves as a visual and physical indication of the consensual power exchange. It can be removed at any time by the Dominant or the submissive, with no ill will, thus signifying a break in the power exchange and a return to equal social standing. It is common that the Dominant partner will set a time period of up to two months around the use of such a collar as a trial period for the dynamic. At the end of the trial period, if both parties are happy with the dynamic and decide to continue, a "training collar" is presented.

The training collar is a personalized collar that is a token of affection and devotion. Accepting a training collar indicates a deepening relationship wherein the submissive is being prepared by the Dominant to serve the Dominant's wishes. Similar to the consideration collar, when worn, the training collar serves as an indication of the power exchange. It's also often used as part of the training. For instance, posture collars are commonly used in order to train a submissive to keep their chin up and show that they are proud to serve. Many people decide to use discreet locking necklaces or fashion collars as training collars so that they do not need to be removed in public. Others choose to only wear their training collars while actively training. Either way, a submissive may ask to be released from their collar (wherein they would return it permanently to the Dominant). Such a break is considered to be more serious and painful for both parties.

Finally, the "slave collar" signifies the deepest level of commitment, and at this point the submissive is considered to be a formal slave, owned by the Dominant. Among some in the BDSM community, this type of collaring involves locking collars or piercings that are only able to be removed by the Dominant, thus seen as a permanent form of bondage for the length of the relationship, unless the Dominant decides to release the slave for an exceptional reason. Many couples that get to this stage in their relationship choose to hold a formal collaring ceremony in order to celebrate the landmark.

Usually, in public play settings, the donning of a collar is an indication that an extra stage of negotiation with a Dominant party is required before others can engage with the submissive. By wearing their Dominant's collar, a submissive is figuratively bound to them, whether literally tethered by a leash or not. It is widely accepted within the BDSM community that if someone is wearing a collar, they are considered to be the private property of whoever affixed the collar. This means that if you see someone wearing a collar in a play setting, you should ask about its connotation before asking them to play.

If you are attending a play party and want to indicate that you're interested in engaging in a submissive role, wearing a collar is not a bad option, but it might create some confusion due to the reasoning stated above. In this case, a casual fashion collar would be suggested over a formal locking collar.

## Body Harness

Body harnesses are an intricate series of straps and handles that wrap around the body in a weblike fashion. Standing alone, they are not intended to restrain a person, but rather to apply pressure over the bound area and produce a feeling of being held. Based on where the lines of the form cinch or frame the body, different styles can objectify and highlight body parts in a particularly lovely manner. Some body harnesses include a strap that runs through the legs, adding genital stimulation or restriction to the smorgasbord of sensations.

Body harnesses also provide attachment points for other

bondage devices such as leashes or straps. Their versatility allows them to be used with or without additional restraint, making them a good item for a variety of activities. For instance, wearing a body harness while doing grocery shopping or house chores can remind a submissive of their Dominant's desires, but allow them to move about freely. If said chores are completed to the Dominant's satisfaction, the harness can be altered to restrain or even suspend the submissive in the air while rewarding them.

Unlike a collar, a body harness is seen as more of a utilitarian form of costume bondage rather than one with meaningful symbolism. Therefore, it might be a better option to wear for flagging submissive tendencies when attending fetish parties. It certainly works just as well as a collar to attach a leash to!

Due to the recent surge of interest in BDSM in the popular culture scene, body harnesses have experienced a fashion resurgence. Be sure to use leather or rope harnesses if you want them to be functional, as the elastic ones meant for fashion purposes aren't as sturdy.

## Corsets

The corset is perhaps one of the most controversial forms of costume bondage in terms of how it affects one's health. While the aesthetic function of the corset has changed over time—sometimes used as a chest binder for a flat look, sometimes to give curves via tightening—the corset has always been used as a shape-shifting device. Due to the solid structure and firm pressure that it provides, when used properly and with moderation, the corset has been known to provide health benefits such as improved posture and anxiety reduction. When it is used to excess, corset wearers experience displaced ribs, lung constriction, organ displacement, and fainting spells, making them fashion victims in the truest sense of the term. Thankfully, due to its popularity over such a long span of time, the corset has gone through many revivals in the fashion industry and has evolved in terms of materials, patterns, and lacing techniques in order to make them healthier to wear.

To safely obtain the hourglass figure long fetishized by the fashion industry, corset enthusiasts are encouraged to slowly build up waist reduction through the techniques of "tight lacing" or "waist training." Tight lacing involves using different increments of waist reduction from one to four inches for short lengths of time, and is best done sparingly, only for performances and other special events.[68] When using this technique, it is recommended to begin with light lacing and work your way up toward a larger waist reduction over time.

| Light lacing | 0-2" reduction | Very light compression |
|---|---|---|
| Moderate lacing | 2-4" reduction | Snug |
| Tight lacing | > 4" reduction | Challenging but comfortable |
| Overlacing | | Anything that hurts, a sign to unlace |

68 "Waist Training vs Tight Lacing—What's the Difference?" *Lucy's Corsetry* (blog), October 13, 2013, https://lucycorsetry.com/2013/10/13/waist-training-vs-tight-lacing/.

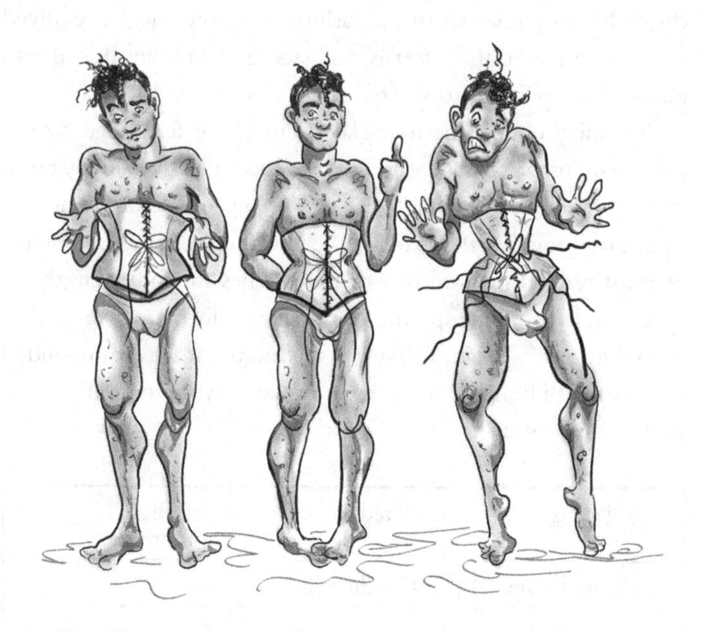

Waist training is a more long-term commitment. Like marathon training, waist training involves consistent, often daily use of a corset toward an end goal of reducing one's natural, uncorseted waist. There are many methods for waist training, so when embarking on a waist-training journey, it is recommended that you heavily research training regimens and figure out which one works best for you. Be sure to consult with your physician and expert resources such as Lucy's Corsetry (www.lucycorsetry.com) for pertinent information.

Despite whether the intended outcomes for corset wearing are short-term or long-term waist reduction, the immediate effects of wearing them are similar. The objectification of the form, constriction of the torso, and movement restriction are all elements that make the corset a wonderful tool for costume bondage.

## Ballet Boots

While all high-heeled shoes present mobility challenges of some kind to novice wearers, the ballet boot is a specific form of fetish footwear intended for bondage. Like many other forms of fashion bondage, the purpose of the ballet boot is twofold: to objectify the foot by forcing it into an aesthetically approved shape and, in doing so, to restrict movement. A slender slipper-shaped foot has long been seen as the feminine ideal, as demonstrated both by the Chinese foot-binding tradition and typical ballet shoes. Like most other types of costume bondage, this slender form does not come without a cost. This is achieved by restricting the wearer's feet to a position en pointe, like a ballerina, which pitches all of the body's weight onto the tips of the toes. Ballet dancers know that moving in this position requires a great deal of built-up ankle strength. Therefore, ballet boots with reinforced ankles are helpful for those who wish to be able to walk.

Ballet boots without reinforced ankles are considered to be of lesser quality and are not intended for prolonged periods of standing or walking. Often, they cannot be used for standing at all. Instead they turn the foot into a fetish object, meant to be adored, admired, and sometimes even worshipped. They also restrict movement. Similar to trying on shoes that are too tight, soon after placing the boots on one's feet, the calves and arches of the foot can cramp. Thus, even with lesser-quality ballet boots, a satisfying degree of masochism and objectification can be explored. If the wearer is not a fan of pain, ballet boots serve as a wonderful invisible leash by discouraging movement. If locomotion in the shoes is desired, arch training along with foot- and ankle-strengthening exercises can help. Additionally, wearing boots with reinforced ankles can help take pressure off the toes, making walking easier.

## Hobble Skirts

A hobble skirt is a skirt with a narrow enough hem to impede one's stride. Strangely enough, the hobble skirt is said to have been inspired by one of the first women to fly in an airplane.[69] At a 1908 Wright brothers demonstration in Le Mans, France, Mrs. Hart O. Berg asked for a ride and became the first American woman to have the privilege of flying as a passenger in an airplane. Mrs. Berg seemed to be concerned about modesty during her maiden voyage, so she tied a rope to secure her skirt around her ankles and prevent it from blowing up in the wind. What she didn't realize was that the way the rope caused her to walk upon landing might be seen as, in the famous words of Neil Armstrong, "one small step for a man, one giant leap for mankind." According to the Smithsonian National Air and Space Museum, a French fashion designer was inspired by the way Mrs. Berg walked away from the aircraft with her skirt still tied and created the hobble skirt based on that now classic "wiggle." Like many other fashion trends, the hobble skirt has gone through a series of deaths and revivals, yet it remains a staple in the bondage community due to its ability to highlight the form as well as restrict movement.

Spanking skirts are hobble skirts that have an opening in the rear to expose the butt cheeks. They prevent squirmy submissives from escaping a spanking scenario easily, and they objectify the rear perfectly to encourage and entice others to spank.

Similar to corsets, hobble skirts restrict movement depending on how tightly they are laced, and it is recommended to slowly build up both intensity and duration when using them.

---

69 "Mrs. Hart O. Berg," *Women in Aviation and Space History* (blog), Smithsonian National Air and Space Museum, accessed September 14, 2017, https://airandspace.si.edu/explore-and-learn/topics/women-in-aviation/berg.cfm.

## Hoods

A hood is a garment intended for the purpose of obscuring the face or even the entire head. Historically, hoods have been worn to protect the head, for warmth, as fashion statements, and for the purposes of maintaining anonymity. In some cases, such as with prisoner hoods, the garments are even used to keep the wearers from seeing their surroundings. Fetish or bondage hoods come in a variety of styles depending on their intended use. For the purposes of dehumanization or depersonalization, hoods that cover the entire face are used. Some versions of these fetish hoods have eye and mouth holes; others completely encase the head. Fashion fetish hoods often leave holes for ponytails, or have built-in wigs for aesthetic purposes. Another style of note is the Sweet Gwendoline hood, which is based off the artwork of John Willie. As you might remember from the chapter on Japanese rope bondage, Willie authored and published *Bizarre* magazine, one of the first bondage magazines in the United States. One of the comic strips featured in the magazine was called *Sweet Gwendoline* and featured a buxom blonde damsel in distress who was constantly finding herself tied up by some villain or another. Gwendoline and her captors were always dressed in fetish gear such as corsets and stiletto heels, and were drawn with overexaggerated curves. The Gwendoline hood encased the entire head and face in leather but for a hole exposing the eyes and bridge of the nose. It was fetishized as an elegant marriage of crude restraint and adorable femininity, and due to its popularity was donned by its namesake character in many cartoons. If you're interested in learning more about fetish fashion, I highly recommend delving deeply into Willie's work. It is a gold mine in terms of the bondage fashion aesthetic and was the inspiration for most of the costume bondage that we see in pop culture today.

## Latex Clothing

Besides leather, latex rubber is the most popular clothing material in the BDSM community. The versatility of the material provides the opportunity to create virtually any type of clothing or accessory, so any form of costume bondage mentioned previously in this chapter can be made from it. That being said, a latex garment does not need to include any sort of restraint in order to be considered a bondage garment. Latex rubber is a bondage tool in and of itself.

The skintight, shiny material hugs every curve of the body in a manner that not only objectifies the body, but also constantly stimulates the skin. The essence of latex is that it becomes like a second skin, encasing the body and creating a new outermost layer. Like many other forms of costume bondage, the tightness of latex garments also creates a pressure on the body that people find to be pleasant and relaxing. The tightness of the garments also necessitates the use of a dressing aid like silicone lube in order to slip them on. Once donned, the friction of the rubber against the body creates a thin film of sweat between the clothes and the skin, which keeps the skin warm and moist. While some find the sweaty sensation to be uncomfortable, many find the wetness and slipperiness that the latex provides to be wildly erotic.

Latex material is relatively thin and easily punctured, so the clothing made from it requires special care to avoid tearing. This provides a unique bondage predicament, as it makes moving about the world, especially sitting in latex, something that requires a bit more mindfulness than the typical garment.

## TUTORIALS

### 1. Collaring Ceremony

Ascribing meaning to specific articles of costume bondage can add a potent layer of meaning to any scene. This is just an example of what I say when I collar my submissives before play. Feel free to be inspired and make your own collar vows!

> Dominant: "With this collar, I am bound to you just as you are bound to me. Until I take it off your neck, I will be responsible for your well-being, and you are to be subservient and obedient."
>
> Submissive: "With this collar, I accept your Dominance and vow to be obedient."

### 2. Rope Body Harness

2.1 Place bight of rope around your partner's neck and measure so that the bight hangs down between their shoulder blades.

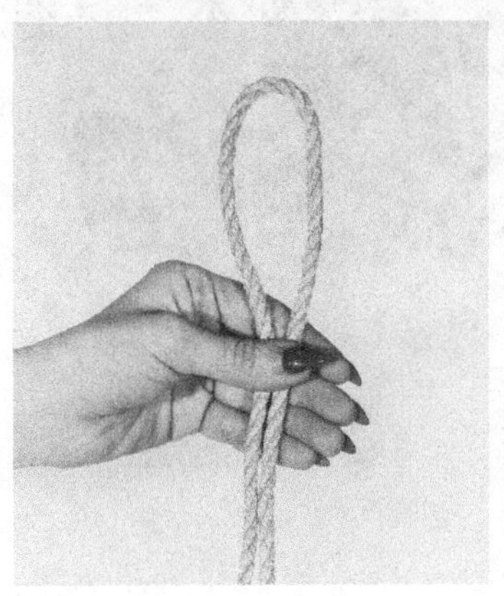

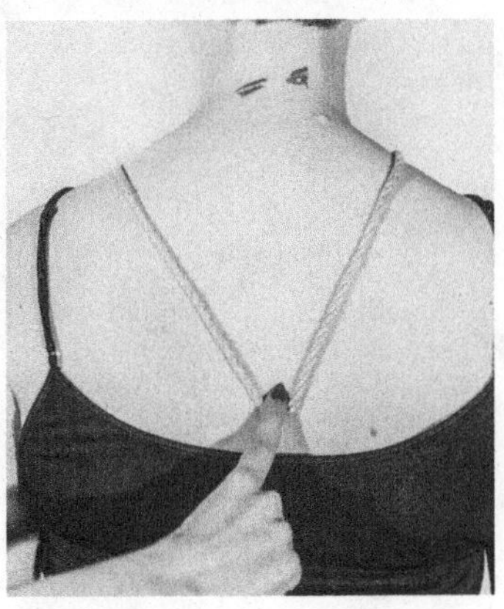

2.2 Tie your knot of choice over breastbone. Two overhand knots will make a square knot that lies flat against the body.

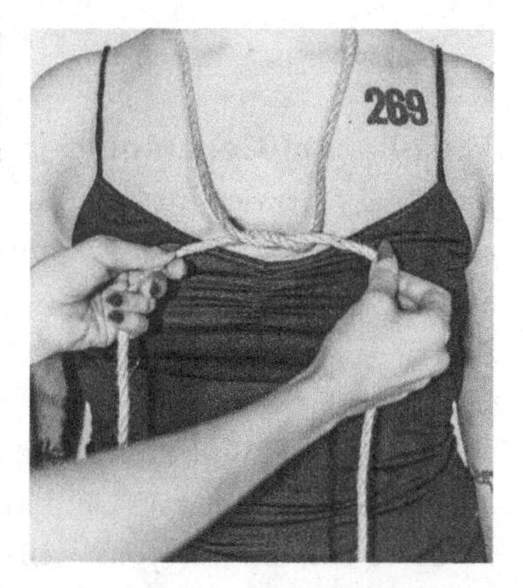


2.3 Twist the ropes around each other, making one- to one-and-a-half-inch twists, not tighter.

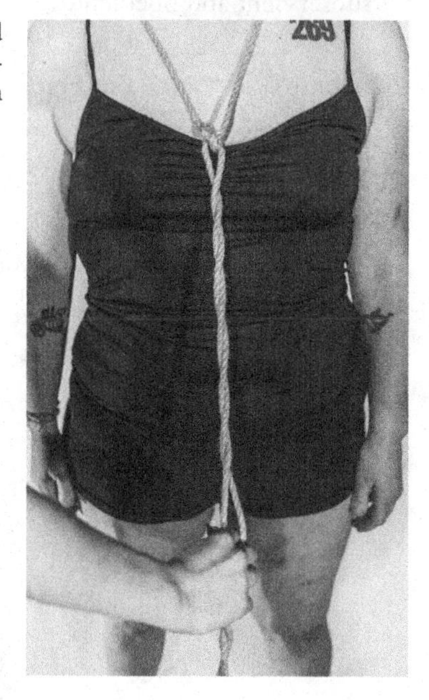

2.4 Pass the ropes between the legs and up through the bight.

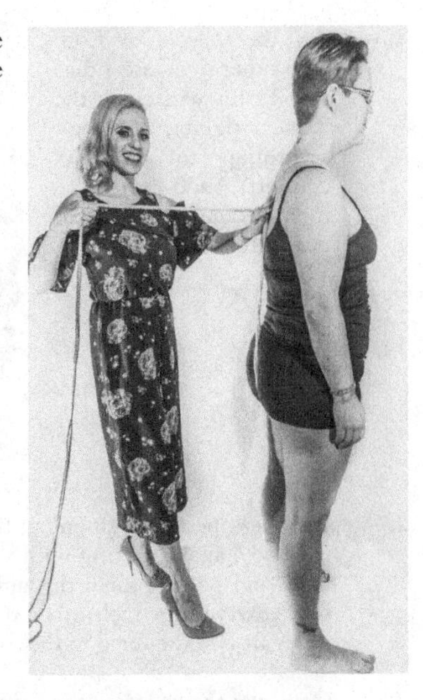

2.5 Split the ropes, bringing them around the torso to the front, and pass the ropes through one of the twists, starting on the side that is closest to the bottom's body, and pulling the ropes through toward you.

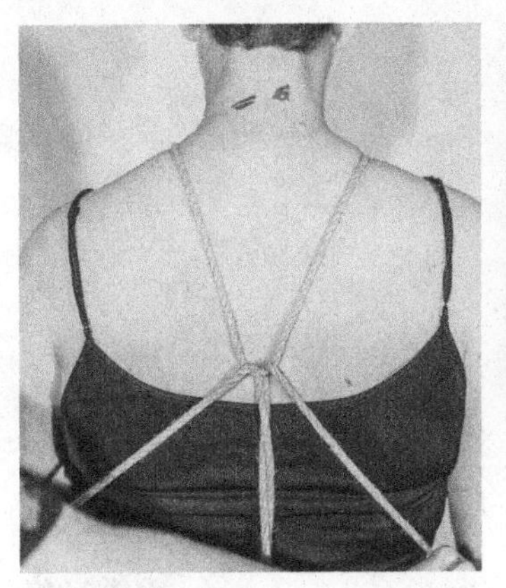

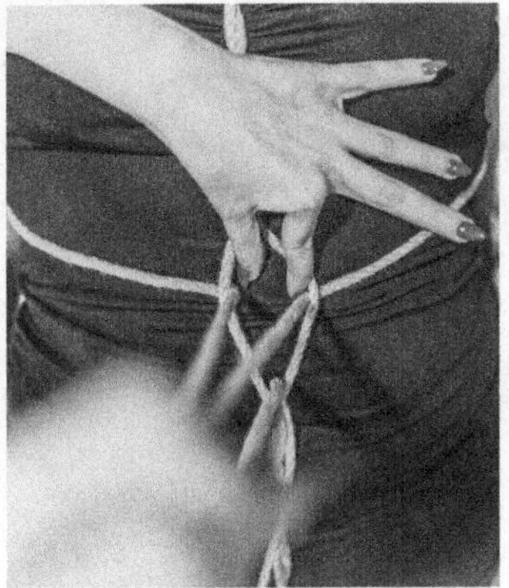

2.6 Pull the ropes away from each other to create a diamond (this will cinch the harness tighter, so adjust according to bottom's comfort), and pass the ropes around the torso to the bottom's back.

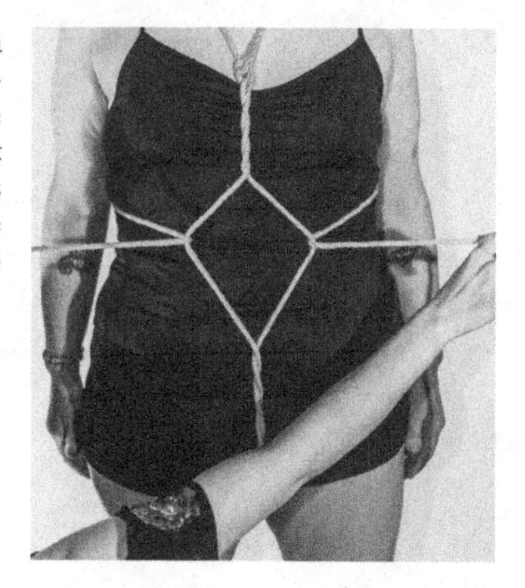

2.7 Pass the ropes through one of the twists, this time at the back of the body, again starting with the rope on the side closest to the body and pulling them through the twist toward you. Pull the ropes away from each other to create a diamond, and pass the ropes around the torso to the front of the bottom's body.

2.8 Continue the process of creating diamonds until you run out of rope or the harness becomes too tight.

2.9 Tie off the running ends to the original bight between the shoulder blades, using the lark's head knot from the tutorial on crotch rope in Chapter 4.

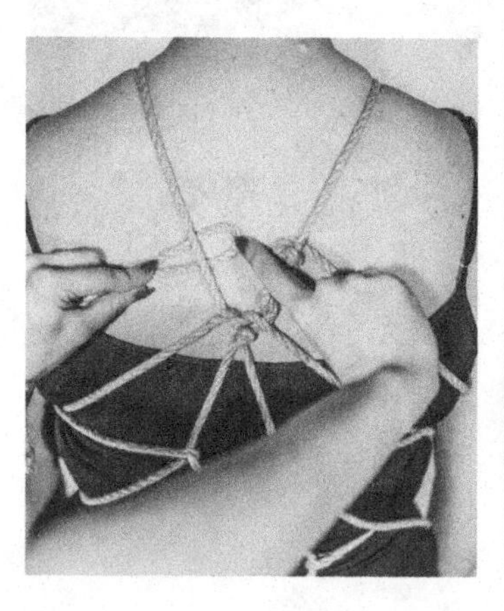

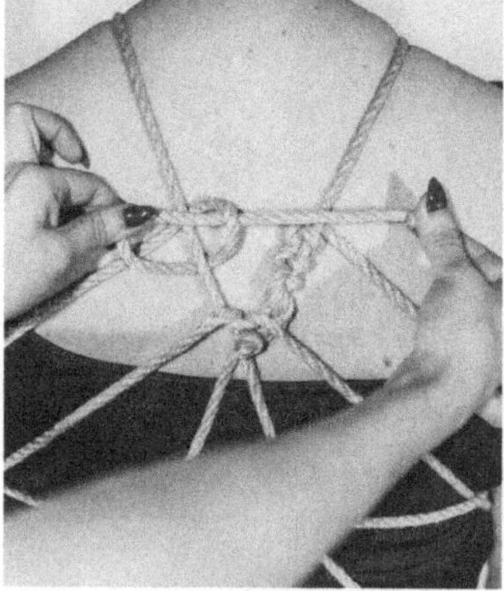

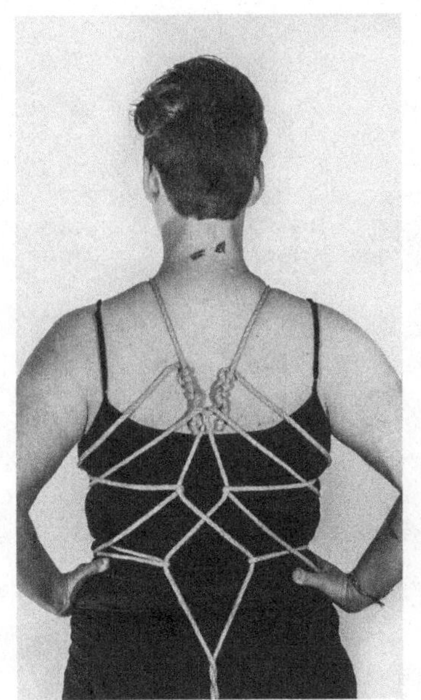

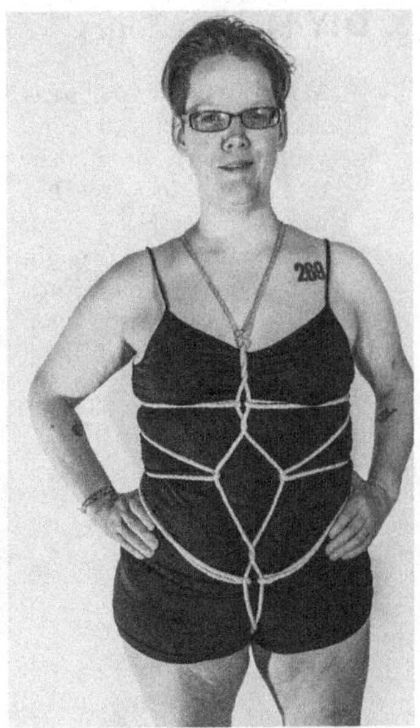

*Bottom: Rocky. Top: Mistress Couple.*

**Safety precautions:** This tie restricts breathing. Make sure that your partner is standing straight with good posture, and that their hands are comfortably at their sides while you are tying, or else their breathing will be even more restricted than intended. Similar to the crotch rope, this tie limits bathroom use, so make sure to allow your partner to use the bathroom before tying it on them.

## 3. DIY Hobble Skirt

3.1 Make sure that your partner has an overhead beam, wall support, or a chair to hold on to while being bound. Have your partner stand up straight with their legs and feet together. Wrap plastic wrap around their waist, down to the ankles.

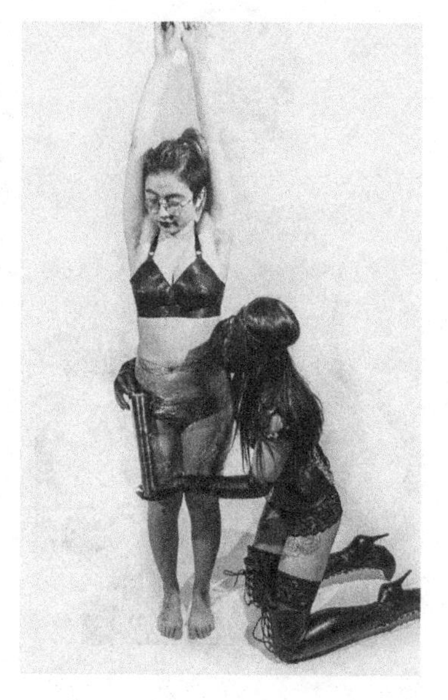

3.2 Tape over the plastic using colored duct tape, making any design or pattern that you desire! Be sure not to wrap too tightly or you will cut off circulation.

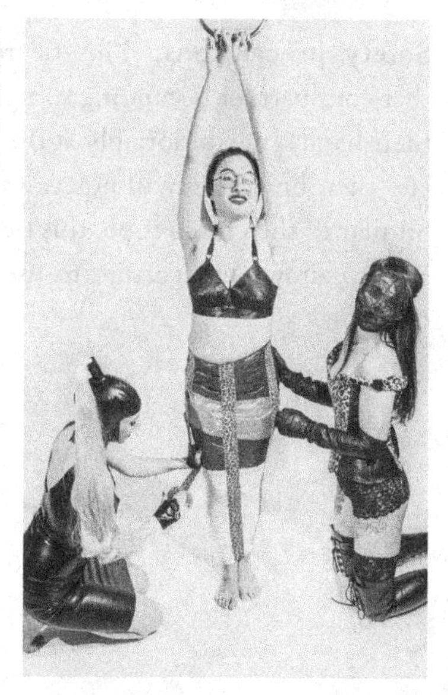

3.3 Cut up the center on the backside of the plastic using safety shears with a rounded edge so as not to cut your partner.

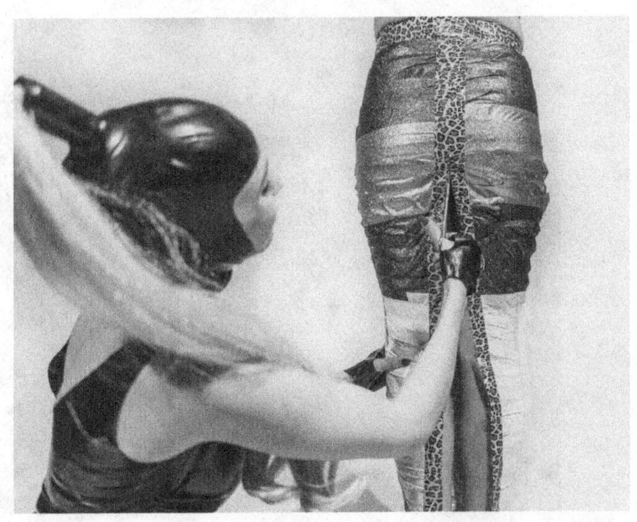

3.4 Mark Xs one inch from the cut on each side, and poke holes through the X marks to create lacing grommets.

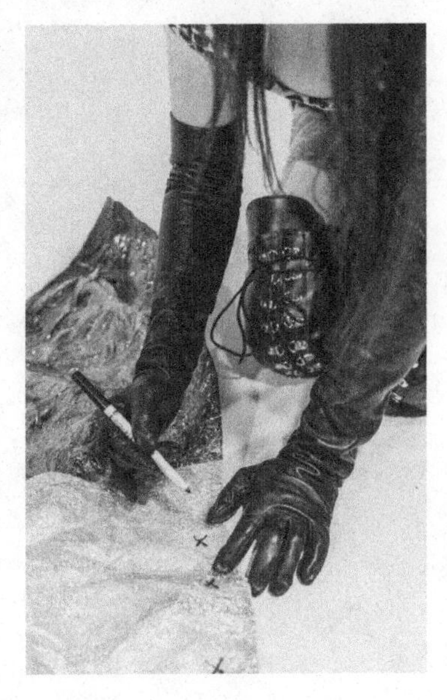

3.5 Hold the newly made garment against your partner's body and thread a ribbon through the holes, tying a bow to secure.

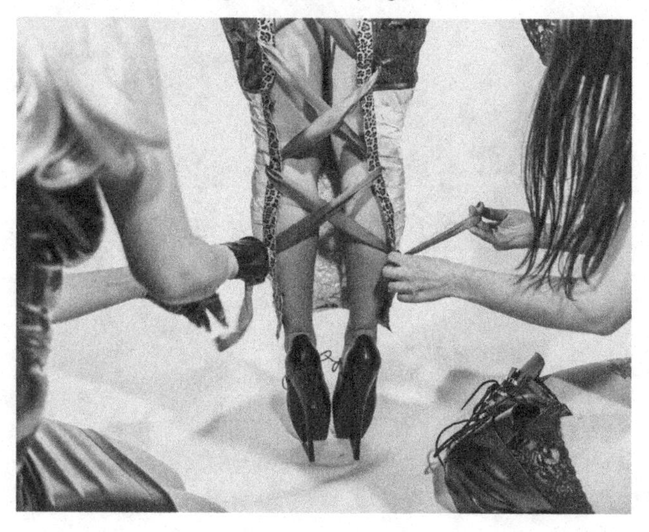

3.6 Make sure that your partner is prepared to take very tiny steps. They'll be your arm candy all night!

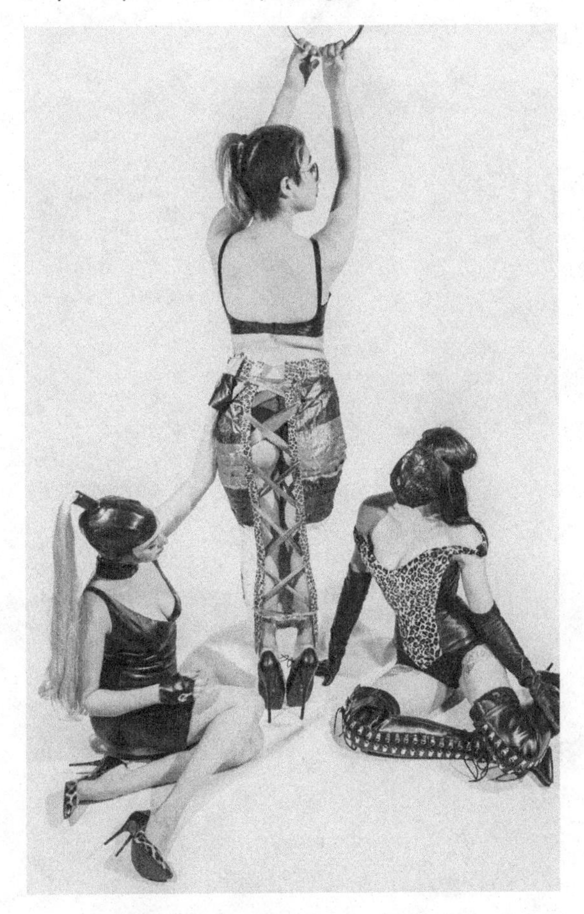

*Bottom: Slice. Tops: Mildred S. Pierce and Mistress Couple.*

**Safety precautions:** Make sure not to cut off circulation by wrapping the tape too tightly. That's really the only danger, besides potentially tripping from lack of balance. You can always tie the skirt more loosely if your partner is having trouble walking.

CHAPTER

8

# SENSATION BONDAGE

We are now entering into new territory regarding the primary focus of each bondage activity. From this chapter on, things get a little convoluted in terms of motivators for participation. Sensation bondage and the other bondage activities explored from here on out focus on a combination of factors (including but not limited to sensory processing, arousal, and facing an ordeal) rather than a single focus (such as restraint). Ultimately, it is up to the practitioner to decide which elements they want to focus on and incorporate those into their practice.

Referring to the chapter on device bondage, you will recall that in addition to restraint, two key functions of bondage are sexual stimulation and torture/pain infliction. It should come as no surprise to you then that there is a form of bondage play that exists primarily for those purposes and views restraint as a secondary benefit. That form of bondage play is called sensation bondage.

Sensation is important because, at our core, we are all beasts. Beasts operate off the information that their senses provide in order to make decisions about the world around them. In today's society, intellect is often valued above sensory awareness. We are encouraged to wear deodorant to prevent us from "smelling bad," most popular foods are laced with chemicals that dull the taste buds, and men in particular are often starved for physical touch. These types of social standards limit us in harmful ways. Without sensory information, the intellect has little to stand on. As you learned at the beginning of this book, our very existence relies on the processing of sensory information that teaches us about our surroundings. In this chapter, you will learn how to recreate some of the sensations experienced during birth through the practice of encasement. But first, you will discover a buffet of new sensations that bondage has to offer, and learn why some people find painful sensations to be pleasurable.

## Flavors of sensation

Sensation bondage typically involves light, pleasing, and often erotic sensations, and is therefore a wonderful gateway into power exchange for beginners. By using the bottom's senses of smell, touch, taste, sight, and sound, a Top can provide a delicious array of sensations. For example, hemp rope has a very distinct smell that can elicit memories of previous bondage experiences and help the bottom to enter into subspace more quickly. It also provides a unique sensation and sound when it is pulled across the skin, as well as an aesthetic beauty that can be appreciated by both partners. While these sensations might be considered to be pleasurable by many, they can easily be modified to suit masochists and those who derive pleasure from painful sensations.

Remember, there are many flavors of sensation, and everyone has their own particular preferences. By adding sensory play into BDSM interactions, Dominants can train their bottoms to be present in their bodies while calming their intellect. This escape away from the mind and into one's body can provide a new lens through which to experience oneself and can be incredibly exciting.

Figuring out what your or your bottom's preferences are through "sensation tasting" can be a lot of fun! We will learn more in the sensory-deprivation chapter about how when one sense is dampened, the others are heightened. For now, we will be focusing mostly on the sense of touch, so tying your partner down and blindfolding them will allow them to enjoy this activity more fully and figure out more easily what their sensation preferences are (plus it's a great excuse to practice what you've learned so far!). If you do not choose to bind your partner for this experiment, it will still work; however, by restraining someone before sensation play, you increase the feeling of vulnerability that charges the scene in an entirely different way. It might be fun to practice this exercise both bound and unbound—you know, for scientific accuracy.

While exploring sensation, you might find that your partner's preferences exist along a spectrum rather than a preference of one over the other. With sensation tasting, much of the excitement comes from creating a wide range of dynamics. You know how some of your favorite songs have a structure that ebbs and flows rather than playing the same note the whole time? Changing volume, time signature, or key midsong is what keeps it interesting. The soft bridge is what makes the loud chorus that much more potent. Using dynamics that oppose each other or build into each other in interesting ways is what you want to strive for in regards to sensation play. You might even want to choose some songs that have interesting dynamics and big climaxes to inspire you to "play along," using your bottom as your instrument.

**Deep pressure vs. light touch:** You learned in the chapter on the birthing experience why deep pressure is a sensation that is enjoyed by most. That being said, light touch can also be very pleasurable. Trying first by dragging your fingers across the skin, determine the amount of pressure that your partner enjoys. Then add a bondage tool to maintain that amount of pressure on the skin once your hand is removed. In this way, the bondage device becomes an extension of your hand. If your partner is someone who enjoys firm pressure all over their body, tune in to the encasement module later in this chapter.

**Rough vs. smooth:** Simply dragging a tool across the bottom's skin can make their hair stand on end. It's a wonderful way to warm up, introduce the implement that you will be using, and awaken the skin. Some bottoms find rough rope such as jute provides a pleasurable scratchy sensation; others prefer the softness and smoothness of silk rope or leather restraints. If you're using rope for this activity, it's imperative to know the burn rate of the rope so as to avoid unwanted rope burns.

**Warm vs. cold:** Wrapping someone in warm rope that just came out of the dryer is a wildly different sensation than locking them in handcuffs or wrapping them in chains that have just come out of the freezer. Cold bondage can be particularly pleasant when it follows impact play, as it can be used for cooling the skin.

**Stillness vs. vibration:** Many genital bondage devices come pre-equipped with vibrators due to the popularity of the sensation. While some find vibration calls attention to the buzzing region in a pleasurable way, others find it to be distracting. Vibration, in conjunction with crotch rope, is often used for forced orgasm play (tying your partner to a device that you know will make them achieve orgasm). Don't have a vibrator? No problem—use an electric toothbrush to create the same effect. It's brutal between the toes for those who are ticklish.

## Masochistic Sensory Experiences

While you might not have flinched or questioned the sensations that were listed above, your reaction to seeing pain listed as a sensation to try might be different. Most of us have a complex relationship with pain because we've experienced it in contexts that we did not consent to or could not control, and therefore many people try to avoid pain altogether. You will discover, however, that just as the sensations above exist on a spectrum, so does pain. There are different flavors of pain (fatigue, sharp, burning, stingy, thuddy, etc.), and if you're experiencing them in a consensual context that involves safewords, you might find that you actually enjoy some of those flavors! If so, welcome to the club—you are a masochist!

Named for *Venus in Furs* author Leopold von Sacher-Masoch, masochism is the practice of seeking the sensation of pain because it is pleasurable. Up until very recently, masochism has been highly stigmatized. *Diagnostic and Statistical Manual of Mental Disorders of the American Psychiatric Association (DSM)* of the American Psychiatric Association viewed masochism as a psychological disorder until 2013, when the fifth edition of the DSM declassified consensual BDSM activities as such. Now, sexual masochism is only referred to as a disorder in individuals who report psychosocial difficulties such as distress or fixation as a result of their activity. In fact, many mental health professionals now believe that masochistic activities can help couples bond and feel at ease due to the production of dopamine and serotonin.[70] Other people liken the headspace that they enter during masochistic play to a runner's high, and this comparison has also greatly helped in destigmatizing it.

Usually, pain is a sensation that is used in addition to the sensations that bondage provides by using impact implements

---

70 Lizette Borreli, "Kinky Sex: 6 Science-Backed Benefits of BDSM," *Medical Daily* (blog), February 10, 2015, https://www.medicaldaily.com/kinky-sex-6-science-backed-benefits-bdsm-321500.

such as floggers, crops, whips, and paddles once the bottom is already bound. That being said, pain can be inflicted through bondage by providing heavy pressure or by physically taxing the body. Knowledge of pressure points and how to use them is very helpful in causing erotic pain, with or without the help of bondage devices. I will not be covering pressure points, as using them requires medical knowledge and advanced technique that should only be employed after intensive study. Without going too far into that territory, I will offer that a study of the traditional Chinese medicine system would help with your exploration. As far as physical taxation goes, any body position is going to become uncomfortable after some time. This type of physically stressful manipulation will be discussed more heavily in Chapter 11. In any masochistic activity, make sure that you're communicating clearly with your partner so that it is hurting "just right" and not pushing them into territory that might be upsetting.

## Pressure and Encasement

Providing a stark contrast to the sensation of pain, encasement is a relaxing form of restraint that provides a sensation of light to medium pressure over the entire body. It may seem contradictory that restraint typically has a calming effect on the body (unless the person struggles with claustrophobia), but remain open-minded; you just learned that in the right circumstances, pain can be pleasurable. It has been scientifically proven that specific types of restraint that are focused on deep pressure or cocooning sensations reduce anxiety. If you think back to the chapter on the wombic experience, you'll see why. This concept was popularized by Dr. Temple Grandin, a professor of animal science and autism spokesperson who is on the spectrum herself. Though not intended to be used in an erotic context, Grandin's "squeeze machine," a deep-pressure machine designed to calm hypersensitive persons using compression, has proven successful in the reduction of both tension and anxiety among children and adults with autism.[71]

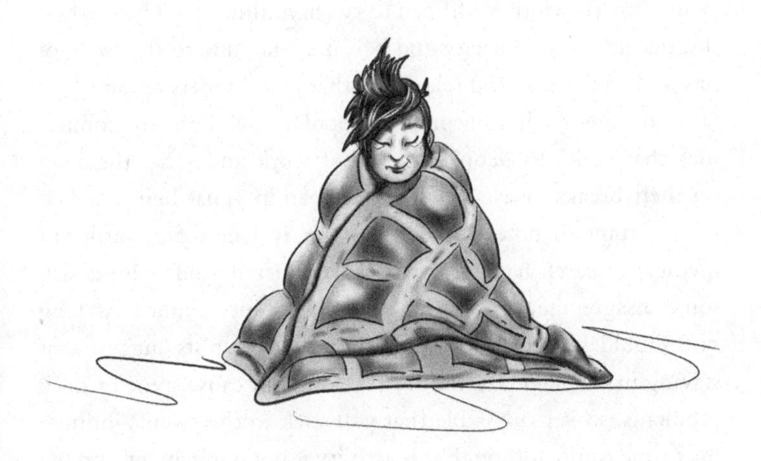

Since its conception in the 1990s, Temple Grandin's approach has been applied to individuals without sensory disorders as well. Weighted blankets have become commonplace in many households because of their comforting effects. The sensation of pressure from the weight of the blanket is known to trigger the release of the neurotransmitter serotonin, a mood enhancer. The blanket's mimicking of a firm embrace may also trigger subconscious memories of being swaddled as an infant, generally the time when people feel most safe and cared for.

Building on this theme, in 2016, Japanese midwife Nobuko Watanabe introduced a method called *Otonamaki*, which directly translates to "adult wrapping." Based on a traditional Japanese practice, *Ohinamaki*, which involves wrapping babies in

---

71 Temple Grandin, "Calming Effects of Deep Touch Pressure in Patients with Autistic Disorder, College Students, and Animals," *Journal of Child and Adolescent Psychopharmacology* 2, no. 1 (Spring 1992), https://doi.org/10.1089/cap.1992.2.63.

muslin cloth, Otonamaki involves being wrapped in a breathable white cloth, lying still in a therapeutic posture (much like the fetal position, but lying on the back), and being held in that posture by the cloth for fifteen to twenty minutes.[72] The method skyrocketed to popularity and became a fad due to the sense of physical well-being and relaxation that practitioners reported. In fact, the activity has become so popular that there are companies that come to people's places of work and wrap them up on their breaks or as after-work recreation. That being said, it is important to note that because this is a new fad, sufficient medical research has not yet been conducted, and there is still some disagreement in the medical community about how long one should be wrapped. Some physical therapists suggest that staying in the fetal position for too long can cause spine or neck problems, so it is advisable that you stick to the twenty-minute max time limit. Although this activity is not publicly interpreted as bondage, the restraint provided by the boundary of the wrapping cloth is undeniable. Visually, it is comparable to examples of encasement that you'll find below.

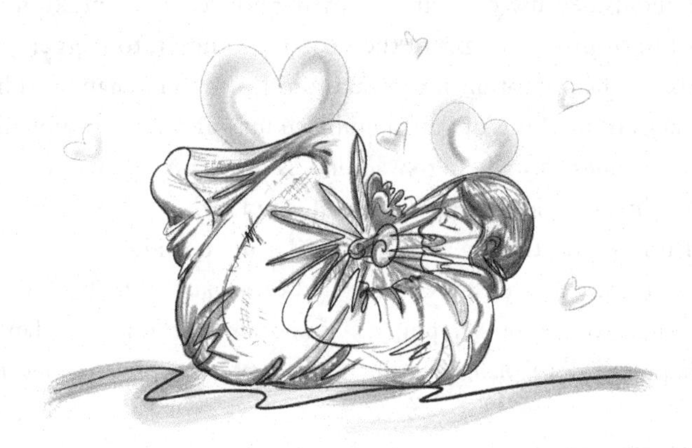

72 Mariko Oi and Yvette Tan, "Why Japanese People Are Wrapping Themselves Up in Cloth," BBC News, December 30, 2016, http://www.bbc.com/news/world-asia-38441166.

In addition to the soothing effects that it creates and the mental vacation that it provides, encasement is often sought out for erotic sensations. Most people who enjoy encasement like to be encased in materials that they fetishize, or at least enjoy on a visceral level. We will discuss fetish items and why they can be such potent tools within a bondage scene in the next chapter. For now, we will simply consider that being encased inside different materials will produce different sensations. First of all, there are different methods for creating the encasement, some (climb-in, wrapping) easier than others (casting). Some materials provide for more stretch, whereas others are more restrictive. Some allow light to penetrate the outer shell; others cocoon someone in complete darkness. Each material has a different smell or texture and a different visual appearance. All of these factors account for varying opinions on which material is the best for encasement. Like most other bondage activities, it's up to you to determine what your or your play partner's personal preferences are.

## Materials for Encasement

**Nylon:** Nylon is highly breathable, at least partially see-through, and very stretchy, so it makes a wonderful encasement material for beginners. Nylon encasement is most frequently participated in by nylon stocking fetishists, who enjoy the sensation on their legs and want to experience it all over their bodies. Total encasement can be achieved by donning multiple pairs of queen-size nylon stockings at once and using the legs of the stockings to secure and tie the bottom into them. There will be a tutorial on how to do this in Chapter 9. A simpler option is to buy a giant nylon body stocking. They're available for purchase online and can be found by searching the terms "Full Body Stocking" and "Encasement" together. Nylon provides a seductively smooth sensation on the skin. It is also very visually and metaphorically stimulating, as it acts as a thin veil between Dom and sub.

**Plastic/vinyl wrap:** Cling wrap is one of the most popular encasement materials due to its availability and affordable price. It is also surprisingly durable! When encased inside a cling-wrap cocoon, it is incredibly difficult to move. There is some stretch to the material, so adding duct tape on top of the plastic like we did in the hobble skirt exercise in Chapter 7 will help to make it more restrictive. Be careful, though, as this also adds more pressure. Communicate with your partner to make sure it isn't too tight. Plastic against the skin almost always causes people to sweat, so be aware of that. If you want to avoid sweating altogether, plastic wrap is not the encasement material for you. For more durable bondage, vinyl pallet wrap is the way to go. In the vanilla world, it is used for industrial purposes and comes in a variety of different gauges that are weight tested. With the proper technique, experienced riggers like Lew Rubens (who invented the technique) can perform suspensions with these materials.

**Latex or balloons:** Latex is a material that is often used for encasement because of the luxurious texture and the pressure that it provides on the skin. You might remember from the chapter on costume bondage that latex does cause sweating, so this is another material to avoid if you don't like that! Though mostly used for sensory deprivation and mummification, which will be discussed in Chapter 10, latex "sucky beds" or vacuum beds provide a wonderfully shrink-wrapped sensation, which could be considered encasement. That being said, these contraptions are very elaborate and quite expensive. Giant balloons are a much more affordable way to achieve the same effect. Plus, in addition to a deflated tight encasement, they provide a unique inflated encasement experience that is strangely evocative of being in the womb. Weather balloons or fetish balloons with a seventy-two-inch diameter are ideal for this type of encasement. You'll need a leaf blower to inflate the balloon and keep air circulating while your partner is inside, and unless you're a seasoned balloon fetishist, you'll probably need some friends to help get your partner in and out of the balloon safely. Balloon encasement is one of the hardest encasements to pull off correctly, but the payoff is worth the effort (especially if your partner is a balloon fetishist). Honestly, balloon encasement might be my absolute favorite form of bondage, and I want you to be able to experience it, so follow the instructions below!

## TUTORIALS

### 1. Modifications for pain

Adding bottle caps, jacks, or spikes underneath rope can make even the most innocent decorative bondage into a torturous experience very quickly!

**Safety precautions:** These little additions will tighten the rope, so the pressure will cause skin indentations and possibly bruises on the body.

### 2. Adult swaddling

2.1 Spread out a sheet and have your partner sit in the center of the sheet in a cross-legged position.

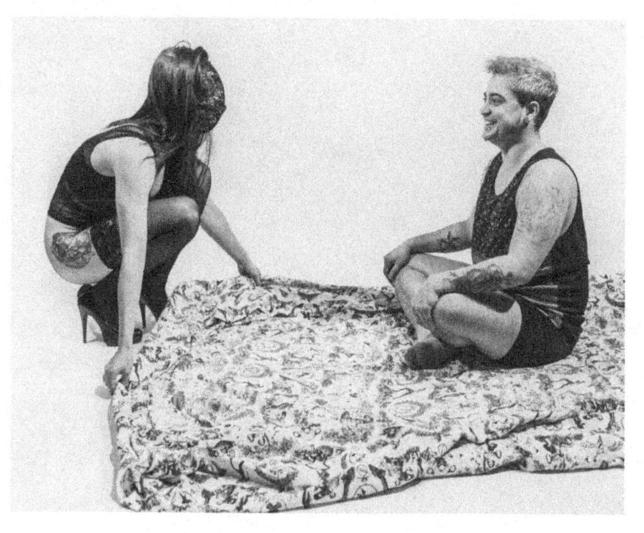

2.2 Place a neck pillow or towel around the neck of your partner.

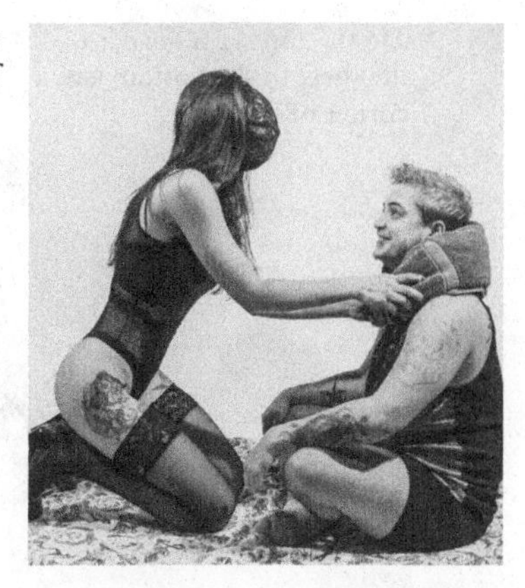

2.3 Pull sheet up over the head of your partner, and fold it back two inches to form a headband around their face.

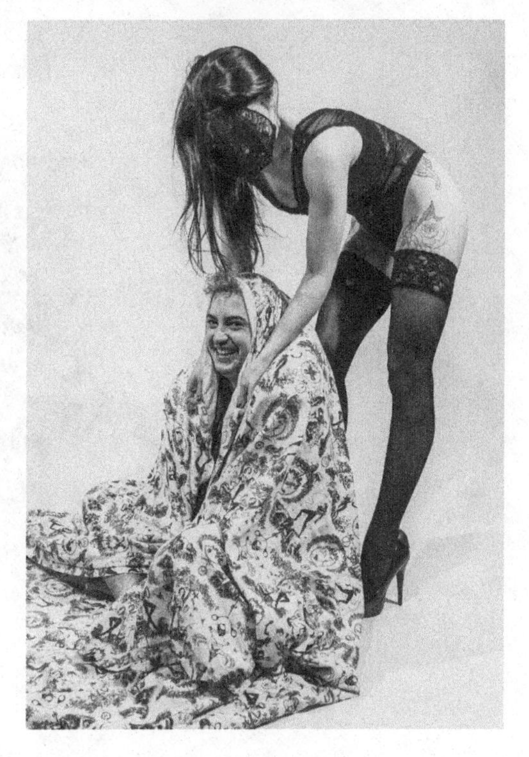

2.4 Tie the top right corner of the sheet to the bottom left corner of the sheet.

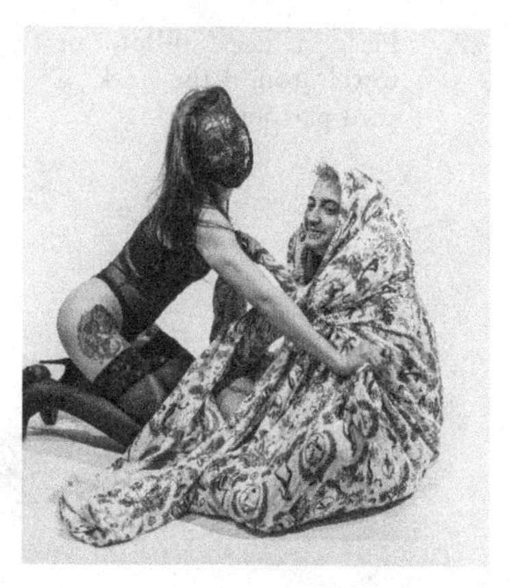

2.5 Tie the top left corner of the sheet to the bottom right corner of the sheet.

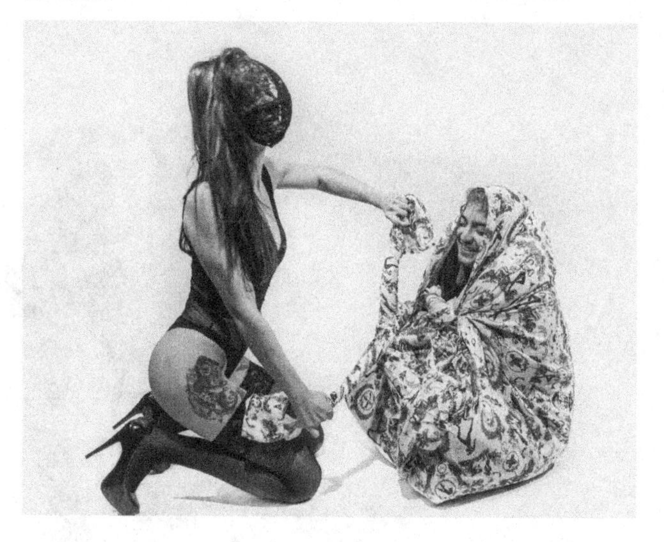

2.6 Help your partner roll onto their back.

2.7 Let them decide if they want to rock themselves, be rocked, or lie still.

2.8 To release, simply untie the sheet corners.

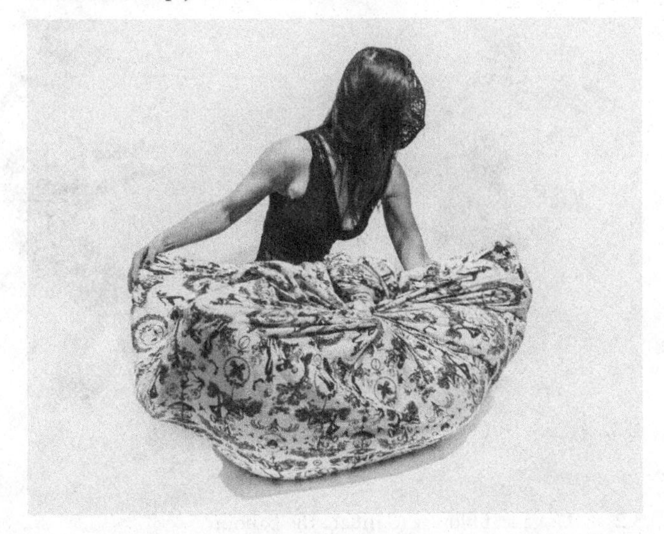

*Bottom: Gage. Top: Mildred S. Pierce.*

## 3. Balloon Encasement

3.1 Stretch the entire balloon, especially the neck of the balloon, as much as possible.

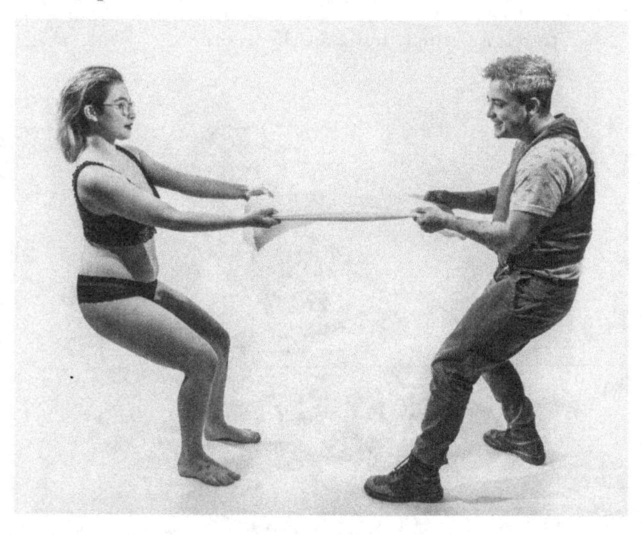

3.2 Use a leaf blower to inflate the balloon.

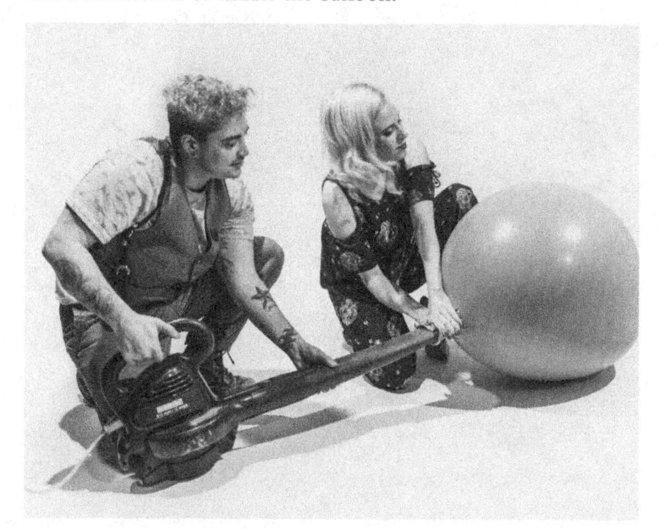

3.3 With two people holding the neck closed, have the bottom align themselves near the neck in a diving position (arms over head).

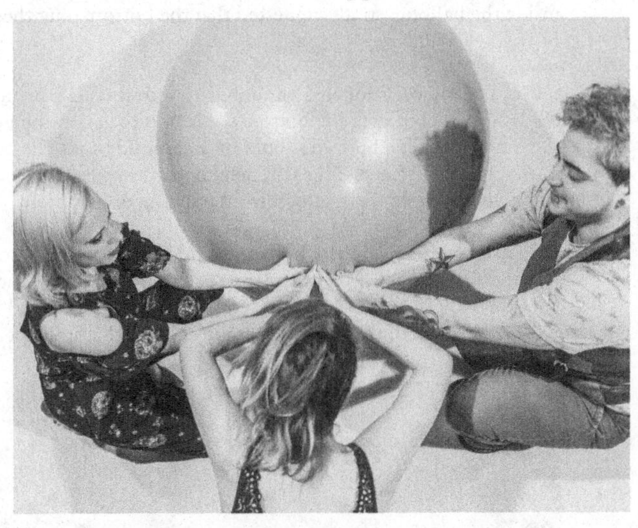

3.4 On the count of three, the balloon holders should stretch the neck open, and the bottom should dive into the balloon up to their chest. This will stop the balloon from deflating.

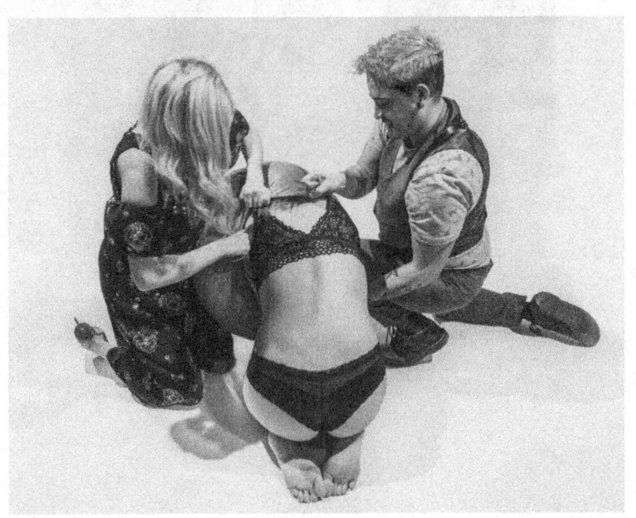

3.5 Stick the leaf blower underneath the seal (against the bottom's back) and inflate the balloon more. This step can be very loud inside the balloon, so it's suggested that the bottom plug their ears or wear earplugs.

3.6 Once the balloon is inflated enough, count to three again and pull the balloon down over the bottom's feet, and then continue inflating it with air. The bottom should move around inside the balloon until it is fully inflated. This will help the airflow inside the balloon and help to prevent the balloon from popping prematurely.

3.7 For ease of breathing, the bottom should position their body so that their head is sticking out of the neck of the balloon. Then deflate the balloon. This creates a wonderful latex body bag! Don't worry, the neck of the balloon is wide enough that it won't choke the bottom.

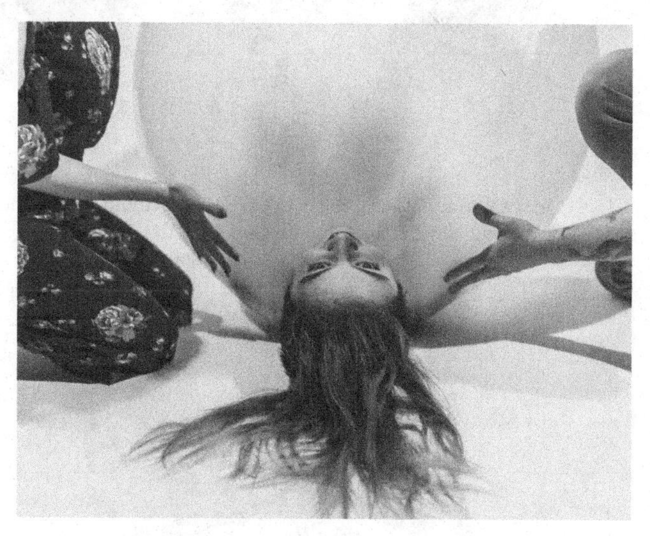

3.8 To get out of the balloon, reinflate it and climb out, or in case of an emergency, cut or pop the balloon.

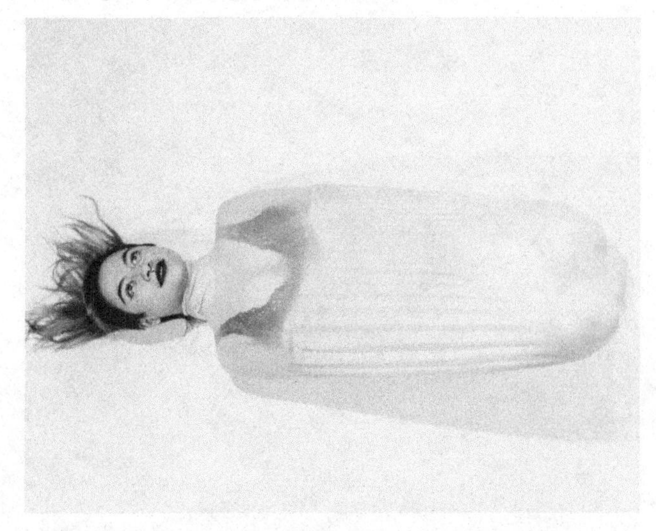

*Bottom: Slice. Tops: Mistress Couple and Gage.*

**Safety precautions:** Make sure that your partner does not have a latex allergy before engaging in this activity. Use earplugs to lessen the possibility of hearing damage. If the balloon is deflated before the bottom can get their head out of the neck, it's possible that their breathing will be obstructed. Because the neck is still open, there will be oxygen flow inside the balloon, albeit limited. Some people do not mind this sensation, but if your partner is claustrophobic, they will not enjoy it at all. Make sure that you have safety shears nearby in case you need to perform a b-section (balloon section)!

CHAPTER

# 9

# FETISH BONDAGE

You just learned about the variety of sensations that bondage can provide and why encasement can be so enjoyable. Similarly, fetishes are generally created because of the pleasurable sensations that they produce. Unfortunately, due to misconstruction by the media and pop culture, fetishes are incredibly misunderstood. This chapter will aim to destigmatize the taboo subject of fetish bondage by explaining what a fetish is and how common it is to have one. It will also discuss the prevalence of different fetishes and the ways in which fetish objects can be used to create the ultimate bondage experience for a partner who considers themselves to be a fetishist.

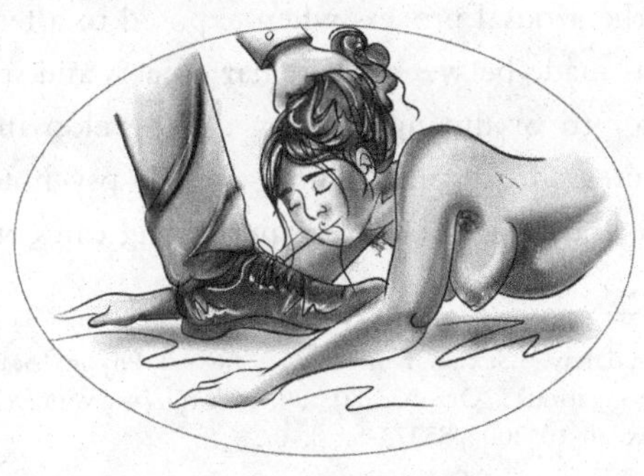

## What Is a Fetish?

*Fetish* is a word that you hear thrown around a lot since BDSM activities entered the mainstream consciousness, but do you actually know what one is? The word *fetish* derives from French, Portuguese, and Latin words meaning "spell," "artificial," and "to make," respectively. Though today people use the word *fetish* to refer to a sexual desire or activity, historically it refers to a single object to which power or value is ascribed. The object becomes empowered by association, which is why there is the notion that the power is supernatural, or somehow artificial. Some of the earliest fetishes were religious idols or ritual objects made from stone. Though believed to possess metaphysical powers that could affect fertility, these fetishes were not implicitly sexual. The idea of sexual fetishism wasn't popularized until the late 1800s, when psychologist Alfred Binet (most noted in the psychology community for the Stanford-Binet intelligence scale) coined the term to refer to the aroused admiration of an inanimate object. Then, in the early 1900s, the term was expanded by Richard von Krafft-Ebing to include body parts that were empowered through sexual association.[73]

No cause for fetishism has been conclusively established by psychologists, but it is widely believed that it likely has something to do with classical conditioning. What that means is that, just as your brain has been trained to make your mouth salivate when you smell your favorite food, it can also be trained to initiate the arousal process when exposed to a fetish object. Associations made between particular objects and sexual stimulation prior to or during puberty can develop into fetishes through increased exposure. There are also psychologists who subscribe to the idea that sensory processing can contribute to

---

73 Dmitry Sudakov, "Sexual Fetishism: A Sexual Physic [sic] Disorder or Harmless Fixation?" October 30, 2006, http://www.pravdareport.com/society/sex/30-10-2006/85273-fetish-0/.

fetishism. In his paper "Phantom limbs, neglect syndromes, repressed memories, and Freudian psychology," Vilayanur S. Ramachandran suggested that the proximity of the sensory processing areas of the brain related to feet and genital stimulation could explain why there are more people who fetishize feet than other body parts.[74]

Other explanations for fetish creation include theories of sexual imprinting during childhood. Though as a society we don't like to think of children as sexual beings, children are curious about and do engage in sexual activity on their own. Fetishism can result when a child has their first experiences with arousal and desire and then associates arousal with whatever stimulus triggered that arousal. This is nothing to be ashamed of. Because they have not yet developed the language to attach to everything, children experience the world on a very sensory level. Enjoying the appearance of an object, the smell of it, the feeling that it creates against the skin, or a combination of all of the above to the point that one experiences pleasure or arousal is actually one of the many joys of life! Ascribing judgment to these behaviors is one of the main things that makes them problematic. Many people end up hiding their fetishes because they have been shamed or told that what they're doing or feeling is wrong. Fetishism can also become problematic when somebody becomes fixated on an object.

Though not scientifically proven, as a fetish provider, I have found that the earlier the exposure to the fetish object, the more likely a fetishist is to be fixated on it. Similarly, the more often the fetishist reinforces the fetish by sexually engaging with the object, the more fixated they become. When someone becomes fixated, it is difficult for them to become aroused without the

---

74 V. S. Ramachandran, "Phantom limbs, neglect syndromes, repressed memories, and Freudian psychology," *International Review of Neurobiology* 37 (1994), 291-333, https://www.ncbi.nlm.nih.gov/pubmed/7883483.

fetish object (direct interaction or fantasizing). As an example, I had a client who fetishized a brush that he was spanked with as a child. This individual experienced his first sensations of arousal during his spankings, and he became very attached to the brush. By the time he brought it to me, he had owned the brush for sixty years and had little interest in sexual scenarios that did not involve it. In this light, many fetishists actually consider their fixation on a fetish item to be a form of sexual or mental bondage, as it can be difficult to disassociate from.

When employed with moderation, sexual fetishes are considered to be completely acceptable components of arousal. It is only when the fixation on fetish objects causes significant stress or has negative effects on a person's life that engaging with a sexual fetish is considered to be a mental disorder.[75] As I stated before, fetishism can also become problematic when people are shamed for engaging in it, and a diagnosis of mental instability does just that. Sexologist Odd Reiersøl has suggested that people who struggle with controlling fixation or unhealthy behavior instead be diagnosed with an impulse-control disorder.[76]

Because shame and stigma often push fetishists into the shadows, we know very little about the prevalence of fetishes in today's society. What we do know is that there are more male-identifying fetishists than female-identifying fetishists.[77] Every few years or so, studies come out with different results as far

---

75 "DSM5: Understanding Fetishistic Disorder," *Hypersexual Disorders*, June 14, 2013. https://www.hypersexualdisorders.com/hypersexual-disorders/dsm5-understanding-fetishistic-disorder/.

76 Odd Reiersøl, PhD, and Svein Skeid, "The ICD Diagnoses of Fetishism and Sadomasochism," *Journal of Homosexuality* 50, no. 2-3 (2008), 243-262, https://doi.org/10.1300/J082v50n02_12.

77 Samantha J. Dawson, Brittany A. Bannerman, and Martin L. Lalumière, "Paraphilic Interests: An Examination of Sex Differences in a Nonclinical Sample," *Sexual Abuse*, Volume 28, Issue 1 (2016), 20-45, https://doi.org/10.1177/1079063214525645.

as the percentage of people purported to fantasize about fetish items, and those self-reported numbers have tended to increase over time. I'd like to think that as society progresses and the shame surrounding fetishism dissipates, those self-reported numbers will become more and more accurate.

My favorite study in fetishism was conducted by an Italian/Swedish research team led by Claudia Scorolli at the University of Bologna. This team downloaded data from hundreds of online fetish discussion groups, which gave them easy access to over five thousand individuals. By going straight to the internet resource rather than inviting people into a clinical setting, Scorolli's team obtained much more honest reporting. Once downloaded, this data was organized into the fetish categories listed below, and then analyzed to determine which fetishes were more common by considering the number of groups devoted to each category, the number of people participating in the groups, and the number of messages exchanged about each fetish.

- A part or feature of the body (e.g., feet or body weight), including body modifications (e.g., tattoos or piercings)
- An object experienced in association with the body (e.g., shoes or panties)
- An object not usually associated with the body (e.g., balloons or food items)
- An event involving only inanimate objects (no examples were found)
- A person's own behavior (e.g., thumb sucking or nail biting)
- A behavior of other persons (e.g., smoking or eating)

- A behavior or situation requiring an interaction with others (e.g., role-play scenarios, or even bondage!)[78]

Data from the study demonstrated that most of the sexual preferences or fetishes were directly associated with the human body, or to objects in close association with the body. Supporting Ramachandran's theory about foot fetishes, feet were the most fetishized body part, with 47 percent frequency relative to other categories. As for the objects, stockings were shown to have the highest relative frequency, coming in at 33 percent, followed closely by footwear at 32 percent and then underwear at 12 percent. This mirrors what I have experienced as a fetish provider, as most of my fetish clients love to worship stockinged feet. They report falling in love with nylon stockings while sitting under the dinner table or hiding under their mother's skirt as children. The study also shed some new light on just how many fetishes there are out there. Though only registering with less than 1 percent relative frequency, 150 group members reported fetishes for hearing aids, and two reported fetishes for pacemakers, supporting something long theorized by fetishists themselves: if an object exists, so does a person with a fetish for that object.

Now that you understand what a fetish is and the different types of fetishes that exist, you can probably see why using fetish items for bondage can be extremely potent. For those with fetishes related to body parts, restraining them and teasing with the body part they desire just out of reach will be delightfully torturous. People with fetishes for objects can be restrained with those objects, or, in the most extreme cases, even encased by them. Examples of this include being pinned down by lots

---

78 C. Scorolli, S. Ghirlanda, M. Enquist, S. Zattoni, and E. A. Jannini, "Relative prevalence of different fetishes," *International Journal of Impotence Research* 19. (2007), 432–437, https://doi.org/10.1038/sj.ijir.3901547.

of sharp, pointy high heels, or the many examples of balloon bondage throughout this book. Another very popular type of fetish bondage involves medical casting or bandaging. These types of medical fetish bondage can be very restrictive as well as passable in vanilla society. By using socially acceptable forms of medical binding, partners who have a medical fetish can engage in long-term bondage play and hide in plain sight! While not as publicly passable as medical fetish, the two tutorials below will cover how to use easily sourced materials such as fetishized body parts and clothing as powerful tools for bondage.

## TUTORIALS

### 1. Foot Fetish: Nylon Encasement

1.1 Using queen-size stockings, pull the crotch down over the face of your partner, and stretch it as far down as it will go.

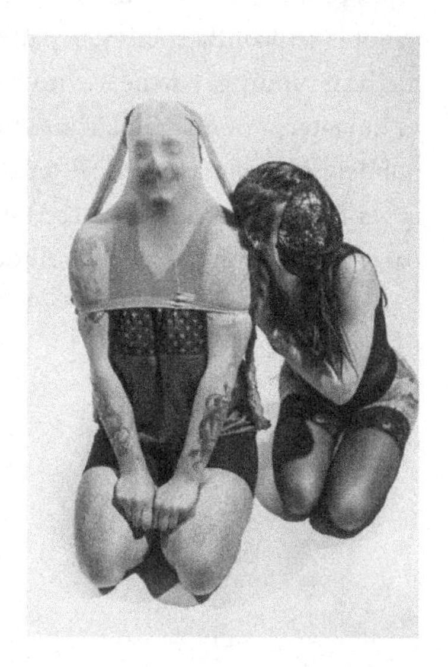

1.2 Use the legs of the stockings to tie your partner's hands behind their back.

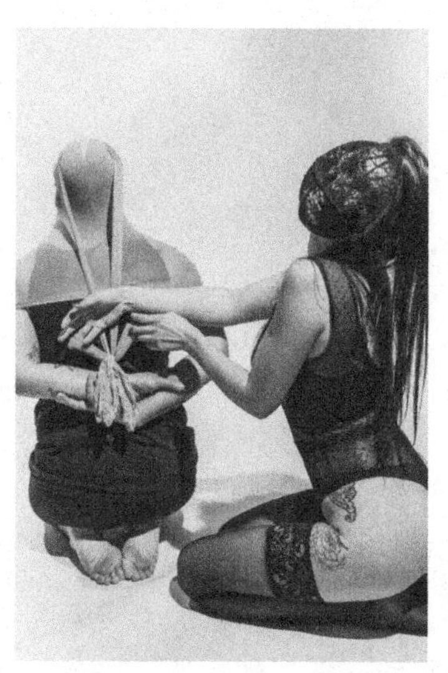

1.3 Put your partner's legs in another pair of stockings, but leave room in the toes so that they can be tied together.

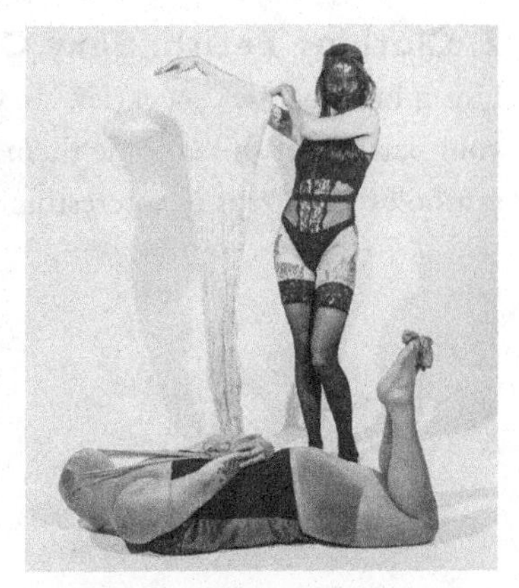

1.4 If you have a full-size body stocking (available at many online retailers), you can use that to fully encase the body. If you position your partner on their stomach and tie the ends of the body stocking together, they will be stuck in a hogtie-type position.

1.5 If your partner has a smelly-foot fetish, you may tie another pair of dirty stockings over their nose. Just be careful not to block the mouth.

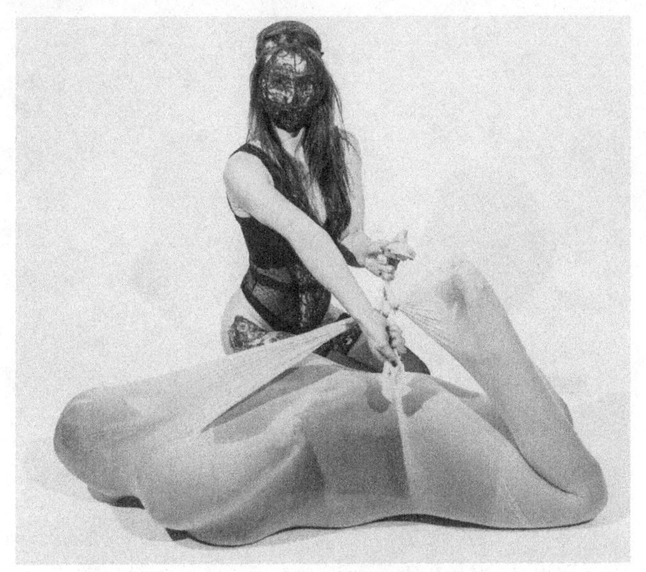

*Bottom: Gage. Top: Mildred S. Pierce.*

## 2. Clothing Fetish: Sexy Clothing Bondage

Using bras, panties, neckties, or whatever other clothing items your partner fetishizes to tie them up can be a lot of fun! Use the armholes and straps in interesting ways—get creative!

CHAPTER

10

# SENSORY DEPRIVATION

Having just discussed the many benefits of engaging the senses, and how they inform our sexual experiences, let's turn our attention to what happens when we limit them or overwhelm them. This chapter will discuss the medical, therapeutic, and erotic applications of sensory deprivation and perceptual isolation techniques. It will also provide you with a list of bondage devices that can be used specifically for sensory deprivation, and even teach you how to make some of those devices out of objects that you can find around your home. First, let's learn what sensory deprivation and perceptual isolation techniques are, and how they affect the body.

Sensory deprivation and perceptual isolation techniques have been used not only in BDSM contexts but also in alternative medicine, meditative practices, and even torture scenarios for years. Deprivation limits the senses by blocking one or more of the receptors (i.e., using a blindfold, or earplugs), whereas perceptual isolation provides a constant uniform stimulus that temporarily changes the way the brain interprets signals. Context and intent are the factors that determine the outcome of a sensory experience.

Short-term sensory deprivation and perceptual isolation, practiced alone or between consenting and caring partners, are most often experienced as relaxing and meditative, but prolonged or nonconsensual sensory-deprivation experiences, such as solitary confinement, are known to result in psychological challenges or even damage. Accounting for personal individuality, the "sweet spot" for BDSM play should be considered to be the overlapping section of a Venn diagram rather than a hard line.

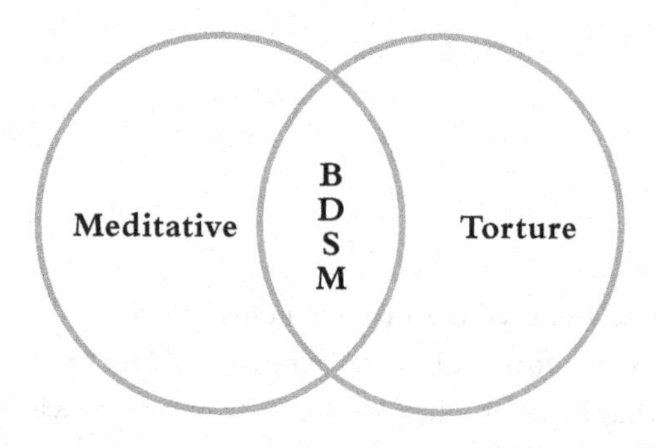


Recalling Chapter 8's discussion about how the senses inform the intellect, it should make sense that consciousness depends on a steady stream of sensory impulses. Building on that train of thought, there is evidence that proprioception (discussed in Chapter 2) also relies on this continuous stream of sensory impulses, not just from outside stimuli, but also from stimuli produced by your brain.[79] When deprived of external stimuli, the brain typically generates its own. These mentally produced sensory stimuli can be described as hallucinations. While many people enjoy these hallucinations in small doses, when experienced for long periods of time they can be disorienting. In this context, it is easy to see how deprivation can be carried into the realm of torture. In situations such as solitary confinement,

79 "Sensory Deprivation." *The British Medical Journal* 2, no. 5003 (1956): 1224-225. http://www.jstor.org/stable/20359926.

for instance, prisoners become disoriented by the deprivation of senses, and become concerned that if they speak, they might incriminate themselves, thus accepting a self-imposed vow of silence. This self-imposed silence interrupts the flow of sensory impulses from within, and paired with the authority-imposed deprivation, contributes to their mental degradation.

In BDSM, it is extremely rare that there be absolutely no stimulus built into a deprivation scenario. Usually there will be an externally imposed stimulus, like a vibrator, or internally projected stimulus, like moans or expressions of gratitude toward the Dominant partner. If you're worried about the deprivation of all five senses being too edgy, you can start with just one by using a blindfold or a gag, and slowly build up. You can also experiment with duration, building up slowly from a few minutes to extended sessions. It's unlikely that heavy sensory-deprivation sessions would extend past a twenty-four-hour period due to the laborious details of eating, voiding, and monitoring, as well as the constraints of everyday responsibilities. With experience and a great deal of careful planning, it is possible to venture into this territory, but know that it is extremely edgy and should be approached with caution.

## Therapeutic Sensory Deprivation

There are two methods of therapeutic sensory deprivation, unrelated to BDSM, referred to as REST (restricted environmental stimulation therapy). Both involve lying or floating on the back in a restful position in a sound-reducing room. In either situation, participants have access to food, drink, and restrooms that are provided in the room, and are also allowed to leave before the designated amount of time has expired. These privileges of personal autonomy in conjunction with the deprivation certainly contribute to having a pleasant and therapeutic experience.

The first method, chamber REST, involves lying on a bed in a fully dark room for up to twenty-four hours. Just imagine—

no cell phones, no music, even! Nothing to distract you, nothing for your mind to latch onto. In the room of darkness, you can simply disconnect. For the second method, called flotation REST, participants float in a tank or pool filled with a solution of water and Epsom salts. The concentration of salt in the water makes the patient buoyant to the point that they feel weightless. I can imagine that this is probably the closest feeling to being in the womb that we can achieve as adults. This type of therapy is usually only recommended for one hour. There are people who like to sleep overnight in flotation REST tanks, but it is unusual for a person to stay in one for twenty-four hours or more. In both types of therapy, movement is restricted by suggestion, but not any mechanical restraints. That being said, it does take major effort to turn over or shift about in a float tank due to the Epsom salt solution, so people generally just stay on their backs for the entire length of the treatment.[80] Both treatments are starting to gain popularity and notoriety, so it is not difficult to find facilities that cater to these services in major cities. Usually, REST sessions will run you about fifty to one hundred dollars per hour, but your money will be put to good use, as the benefits of REST therapy are plentiful.

Chamber REST promotes deep thought, better memory, and elevated mood and reduces stress-related illnesses or behaviors. As such, chamber REST is a wonderful tool for tackling personal vices. Some studies have indicated that, when combined with anti-alcohol education, people who participate in chamber REST are able to significantly reduce their consumption of alcohol.[81]

---

80 Christine Hanchett, "How Sensory Deprivation Isolation Chambers Work," *Examined Existence* (blog), accessed April 15, 2018, https://examinedexistence.com/the-science-of-sensory-deprivation-how-does-sensory-deprivation-work/.

81 Peter Suedfeld and Stanley Coren, "Perceptual isolation, sensory deprivation, and REST: Moving introductory psychology texts out of the 1950s," *Canadian Psychology* 30, no. 1 (January 1989), 17-29, http://dx.doi.org/10.1037/h0079795.

Chamber REST has also been proven to be effective in helping people quit smoking—far more effective than nicotine patches.[82] Due to its high levels of efficacy, practitioners of chamber REST have also explored its use in the treatment of mental disorders with great success. On the contrary, flotation REST is seen as more of a recreational tool. The Epsom salts have a therapeutic effect on stiff muscles, so it is geared more toward use with stress-related disorders, pain reduction, and insomnia.

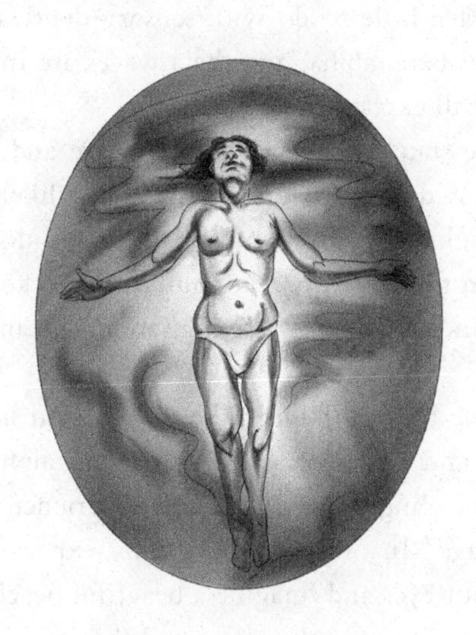

82 Peter Suedfeld and Gloria Baker-Brown, "Restricted environmental stimulation therapy of smoking: A parametric study," *Addictive Behaviors* 12, no. 3 (1987), 263–267, https://doi.org/10.1016/0306-4603(87)90037-2.

## Brain Waves and Sensory Deprivation

In order to understand why these two types of therapy are so effective, you'll need to understand some basics about the functioning of brain waves. There are five different frequencies of wave that the brain is consistently producing: beta, alpha, theta, delta, and gamma. Everything you think, do, say, and feel is regulated by the frequency of your brain waves, and which frequency is dominant in any given situation. Gamma waves and delta waves have little to do with sensory deprivation so we'll skip them, but beta, alpha, and theta waves are intrinsic to the process, so I will explain them below.

Beta is the state in which you are active and alert, so it is most dominant during waking hours. Most likely, while you are reading right now, your mind is in a beta-dominant state. Beta waves, in the appropriate amount, help us keep our focus, concentrate, and finish tasks. Having too much can lead to stress or anxiety.[83]

Alpha is the bridge between the waking and sleeping states, or conscious and subconscious mind. In an alpha state, most people report feeling very relaxed and experience daydreaming and fantasizing.[84] In order to more fully experience an alpha state, close your eyes and imagine a beautiful beachscape. Envision the sun setting over the water and the sound of the waves lapping against the shore. This is the beginning of inducing an alpha-dominant state. Alpha brain waves have been known to lessen pain and are useful in healing, which is why fantasizing feels so good!

---

83 "5 Types of Brain Waves [sic] Frequencies: Gamma, Beta, Alpha, Theta, Delta," *Mental Health Daily* (blog), April 15, 2014, https://mentalhealthdaily.com/2014/04/15/5-types-of-brain-waves-frequencies-gamma-beta-alpha-theta-delta/.

84 "Alpha Brain Waves: 8 Hz to 12 Hz," *Mental Health Daily* (blog), April 11, 2014, https://mentalhealthdaily.com/2014/04/11/alpha-brain-waves-8-hz-to-12-hz/.

A theta state is a very deep state of relaxation. This state is used in meditation, hypnosis, and dreaming and can be induced artificially by listening to tones that resonate in the same frequency. Theta waves are connected to the emotional states that are hidden during everyday interactions. Perhaps they tie into the concept of urami from Chapter 3. They are also involved in restorative sleep, and are typically dominant immediately before falling asleep and upon waking. As long as you don't have an excess of theta waves while awake (which may increase the likelihood of depression), they are very helpful.[85]

During chamber and flotation REST, the brain transitions from a beta- or alpha-dominant state to a theta-dominant state. In many cases, this relaxed state leads to the person falling asleep, though in monitored situations this can be avoided. It is common in both practices for loudspeaker and monitoring systems to be used to awaken participants should they fall asleep. However, it is less likely that a participant will fall asleep during flotation REST, as the unique sensation tends to sustain the theta state. Many people report that the sustained theta state feels like consciously dreaming, and some use it as a tool for boosting creativity, problem solving, or meditative effects.

## Sensory-Deprivation Bondage

We can use the information that we know about therapeutic sensory deprivation and brain-wave patterns to inform our BDSM play. By placing a consenting partner into sensory deprivation, we can shift their perception from one that is focused on active processing to one that is far more relaxed and susceptible to the power of suggestion. Because of this, many people who have

---

85 "5 Types of Brain Waves Frequencies: Gamma, Beta, Alpha, Theta, Delta," *Mental Health Daily* (blog), April 15, 2014, https://mentalhealthdaily.com/2014/04/15/5-types-of-brain-waves-frequencies-gamma-beta-alpha-theta-delta/.

demanding professional or personal lives greatly appreciate the benefits that they receive from sensory deprivation. In these types of situations, the opportunity to shut off the conscious brain and slip deep into one's own subconscious under the careful supervision of a loved one or a fetish provider can seem invaluable. Light sensory deprivation can be used by Tops to gently coax (with permission, of course) their active-minded bottoms into a more submissive state of mind, with the simple application of a blindfold or gag. More advanced applications of sensory-deprivation bondage, such as full-body mummification, can also be used as a form of tease and denial. Generally in these types of scenarios, the entire body is encased in restrictive bondage, but the genitals are left exposed for pleasure or torture. With the rest of the senses deprived, the sensations in the genitals are greatly enhanced.

Finally, potentially the most intense form of sensory-deprivation bondage actually utilizes both mummification and perceptual isolation—a constant uniform stimulation such as flashes of lights or colors, or static sound. Some people use a device called Ganzfeld goggles to create perceptual isolation. While the user is wearing these goggles, their brain becomes confused by the unchanging sensory information, cuts off the input, and often manufactures its own images and sounds. These images and sounds may be thought of as mild hallucinations.[86] Most folks report mild rather than vivid hallucinations while using Ganzfeld devices but find that they are helpful to eliminate excess chatter in the mind. Obviously, hallucination ventures into edgy territory and should only be done under strict monitoring with an experienced partner.

---

86 Jiří Wackermann, Peter Pütz, Carsten Allefeld, "Ganzfeld-induced hallucinatory experience, its phenomenology and cerebral electrophysiology," *Cortex* 44 (November-December 2008), 1364–1378, https://doi.org/10.1016/j.cortex.2007.05.003.

### *Tools for Sensory Deprivation*

**Blindfolds:** Blindfolds are available for purchase in a variety of materials including leather, silicone, and cloth. If you don't have a blindfold, you can easily create one by repurposing a sleep mask, silk scarf, or handkerchief. The removal of vision adds another dimension to power exchange by compelling one partner to rely on other senses for information. Blindfolded play can result in more efficient communication because participants are forced to rely more on verbal or tactile cues rather than visual ones. Blindfolding also has interesting implications for orgasm control. Removing the sense of sight from a partner who is overly stimulated by visual input might prolong sex before orgasm. Removing sight from a partner who is overly stimulated by physical input will do just the opposite, tipping them over the edge of the erotic waterfall and into the throes of orgasmic ecstasy.

**Gags:** Breathable gags are the best for sensory-deprivation scenarios because they permit the passage of air and are less likely to cause choking when worn for extended periods of time. These gags have little holes drilled through them to ensure minimum talking and maximum breathing. It's important that you never use a mouth gag when the gagged person isn't feeling well. Even if it's just a cold or allergies that left them feeling under the weather, a gag should be excluded from your scene. If you're wrapping the face of a gagged person, make sure to leave the nasal passages uncovered, or to use breathing tubes so that the passage of air isn't too limited. If you plan on leaving someone in sensory deprivation for longer than twenty minutes, it might be best to forgo a gag altogether to avoid stressing the jaw. You may still restrict speech by wrapping the face and covering the mouth (as long as breathing tubes are used in the nostrils). As in other situations where speech is restricted, it is imperative that a nonverbal communication system be employed in case the bottom needs to communicate.

**Breathing tubes:** Plastic tubes, drinking straws, and even ziti pasta can be used to elongate the nasal breathing passages and provide precious oxygen to your bottom. Ziti noodles should only be used in short-term bondage scenarios, as the moisture inside the nose can turn them soggy. Nasal tubes slow breathing significantly and reduce the amount of oxygen intake, so bottoms need to be strictly monitored. Similar to gags, bottoms with breathing difficulties spurred on by colds or allergies should not use breathing tubes, as they can be easily blocked and cause suffocation. Breathing tubes are only fun when they work, so make sure to keep your partner breathing at a pace that is comfortable for them. Typically, while fitting a bottom for breathing tubes, you'd leave the hands free and mouth easily unblockable so that they can communicate their ability to breathe comfortably via a thumbs-up or thumbs-down signal. If the thumb moves from upright to anywhere past horizontal, the mouth should be unblocked immediately.

**Earplugs:** Earplugs are useful for drowning out sound. Depending on the level of sound dampening you desire, you can use light plugs made from toilet paper or cotton balls, or heavier plugs made from silicone, which are meant for noise canceling. If you are mummifying the head in plastic wrap or bondage tape, the placement and removal of earplugs is easy, as you can simply move the material aside to access the ears. With the addition of duct tape or full-head hoods, putting earplugs in and taking them out can become quite laborious. They should only be used once you're positive that you've communicated everything that you need to with your partner, and similar to gags, should only be used with the employment of nonverbal communication techniques such as hand squeezing.

**Hoods:** Hoods are a catchall for bondage of the face. As discussed in the costume bondage chapter, there are myriad designs for hoods. While some, like Gwendoline hoods, leave the eyes and nostrils open, isolation hoods completely encase the entire head, blocking out all of the senses. It is recommended that when starting exploration with hoods, you use one that leaves at least one, if not more, of the senses intact. Then, if your bottom is ready and you so desire, you can add blindfolds or gags on top of it. There are even some styles of hoods that include layers, the first layer masking the face but leaving all of the senses open, and the outer layer with a zipper that can close them off individually or all together. This layered effect is particularly interesting for slow, mindful transitions into a sensory-deprived state. Other hoods are fitted with pockets for headphones so that the Dominant can play audio to the bottom while the other senses are deprived. All of the safety precautions that apply to blindfolds, gags, and earplugs also apply to hoods.

**Mummification:** Mummification is an advanced form of bondage in which the bottom is partially or fully cocooned by wraps made from a variety of materials. The process leaves whatever body parts it covers completely restricted and immobilized in its wake. Think back to our hobble skirt exercise from Chapter 7. That tutorial included the basic wrapping and layering techniques needed for mummification—just apply the same techniques to the rest of the body! For an element of sensory overload in conjunction with the deprivation, some skin can be left unwrapped and vulnerable to touch. Usually, people are mummified in a supported standing position (against a pole or piece of bondage furniture), or in a supine position (lying on a bed or bondage table), however, more intricate and difficult positions can be explored for those seeking higher degrees of intensity. It's important to note that the wrapping of the body will cause the bottom to sweat a lot during the process, and will leave them cold and potentially dehydrated afterward, so be sure to have towels and blankets nearby, as well as a squirting water bottle or sippy cup. Safety shears are also a necessary tool for quick and efficient escape. Have a prenegotiated nonverbal safeword, either using hand squeezing or a hum or grunt.

**Sleepsacks and body bags:** Sleepsacks and body bags are often used once someone graduates past basic mummification. Similar to a conventional sleeping bag, a sleepsack is a tube of fabric that can be climbed into and zipped up to the neck. Triple zippers are usually employed to allow for an opening anywhere along the length of the zipper. Usually, sleepsacks are also fabricated with belts to make the sack's fit adjustable. Most people like the fit to be very tight on the body so as to restrict movement as much as possible. Other features that restrict movement include interior arm and leg sleeves. Sleepsacks are often made of spandex, neoprene, rubber, and leather (listed in order from beginner to advanced), each of which have their own set of pros and cons in regards to durability, wear and tear, breathability, and stretch. Because sleepsacks involve a hefty financial investment, as well as physical adjustment, it is recommended that you work your way up from mummification wrapping and sheet mummification before graduating to a sleepsack. The same safeword considerations as with mummification techniques apply to sleepsacks and body bags.

**Latex sucky beds:** As mentioned in Chapter 8 on encasement, latex sucky beds are a special type of body bag used for sensory deprivation. Because sleepsacks are constructed to be formfitting, they typically cannot be used by multiple people unless those people share similar measurements. Sucky beds eliminate this issue—if you have a shrink-wrap machine in your kitchen for storing and freezing food, you can imagine how. Once the bottom situates themselves between two sheets of latex, all of the air is vacuumed out, leaving them stuck, à la Han Solo in carbonite. To allow for proper airflow and breathing, all sucky beds are equipped with either a hole for the head to escape or a breathing tube. Other versions of sucky beds, such as the cube, have been constructed using PVC piping to create a three-dimensional encasement rather than a two-dimensional one. These cubes can actually allow for someone to be simultaneously encased and suspended in midair. Because the latex material feels so much like skin, being suspended and encased in it can create similar sensations to flotation REST. The benefits of sucky beds come with a cost, though. Due to the expense of latex material and the novelty of these devices, latex sucky beds will cost you a pretty penny. They require a great deal of care, because latex can be easily torn or punctured, especially if it degrades from sweat and oils from the skin. Because of this, sucky beds must be carefully washed, dried, and stored between each use, and most people find them to be too high-maintenance for practical bondage. If you're looking to experience a similar sensation without all of the hassle, try the balloon encasement tutorial from Chapter 8.

**Mind machines:** Wearing a blindfold can put the brain to sleep.[87] That's wonderful if it's your intention, but if your goal is hallucination or sensory distortions, the brain needs to stay awake with minimal stimulation. Light and sound mind machines work to guide your brain into a meditative state primed for

---

87 Biotele, "Ganzfeld: Hack Your Brain the Legal Way," Instructables, Accessed Dec 22, 2017. http://www.instructables.com/id/Ganzfeld-Hack-Your-Brain-the-Legal-Way/.

hallucination using synchronized visuals and specialized tones. This process of tuning the brain is called entrainment.[88] Some mind machines use fancy versions of Ganzfeld goggles, which can transmit light indirectly onto closed or open eyes.[89] If the eyes are open, the goggles create the illusion of an infinitely expanding open field of vision. In response to the seemingly blank field of vision, interference patterns from the brain generate hallucinations of kaleidoscopic structures.[90] This psychedelic effect doesn't come without a cost, though. Mind machines can cost anywhere between $200 and $500, so knowing how to hack a Ganzfeld device with regular household items can be useful. Many "mind hackers" swear by placing halves of Ping-Pong balls over the eyes so they can only see diffuse white light, and by playing white noise through headphones or static sounds on the television.[91] The version of Ganzfeld goggles that will be featured in the tutorial section is slightly more elaborate but just as effective as those solutions. Our modifications will make it easier and more comfortable to wear the goggles for extended periods of time.

---

88 Ibid.

89 "The Laxman System," Laxman UK, Accessed Dec 22, 2017. http://www.laxman-uk.com/index.htm.

90 Ibid.

91 Biotele, "Ganzfeld: Hack Your Brain The Legal Way," Instructables, Accessed Dec 22, 2017. http://www.instructables.com/id/Ganzfeld-Hack-Your-Brain-the-Legal-Way/.

# TUTORIALS

## 1. Bedsheet and belt sleepsack

1.1 Measure belts around your partner's body. We recommend using five belts: one around the shoulders, one around the midsection, one to secure the wrists to the waist, one directly above or below the knees, and one around the ankles. If you need to elongate a belt, you can attach two belts together—just make sure that the buckle is not underneath your partner or that will be uncomfortable!

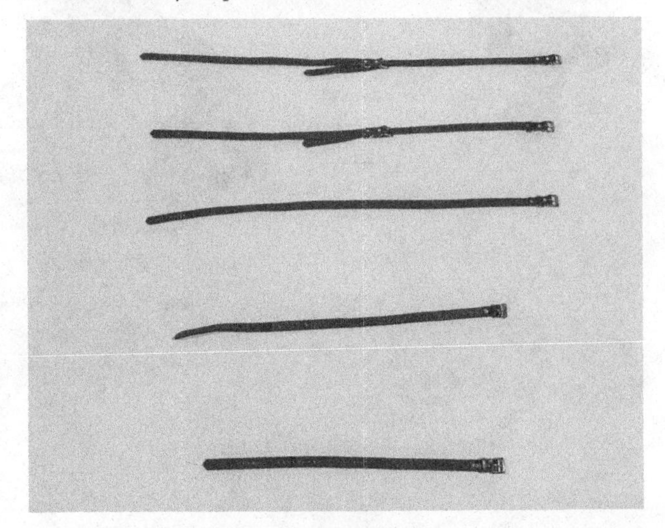

1.2 Spread the belts out in the alignment that they will be used to secure your partner.

1.3 Place a bedsheet on top of the belts.

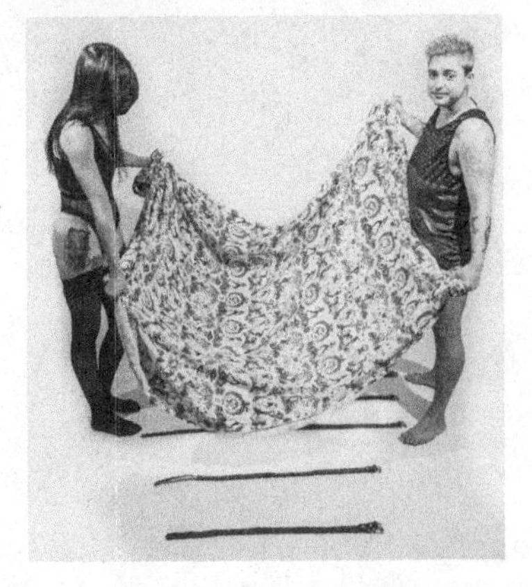

1.4 Have your partner lie down centered on the sheet, with their head sticking out the end (unless they want to be fully encased).

1.5 Tuck the right side of the sheet underneath your partner's body, then do the same with the left side of the sheet.

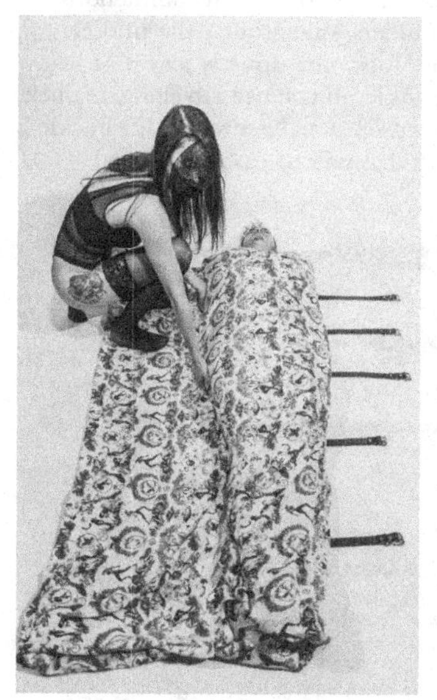

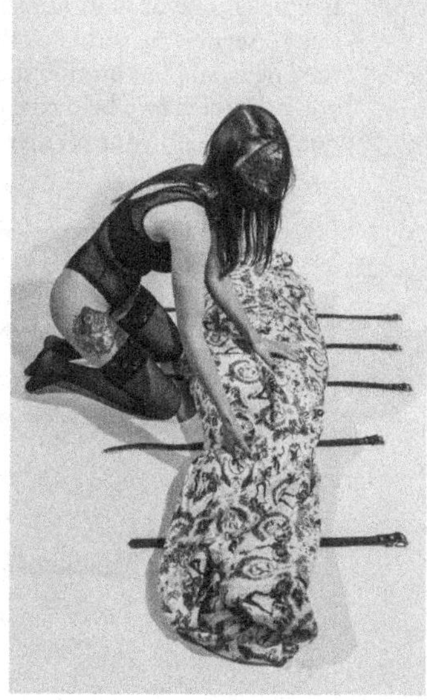

1.6 Secure belts, and voilà!

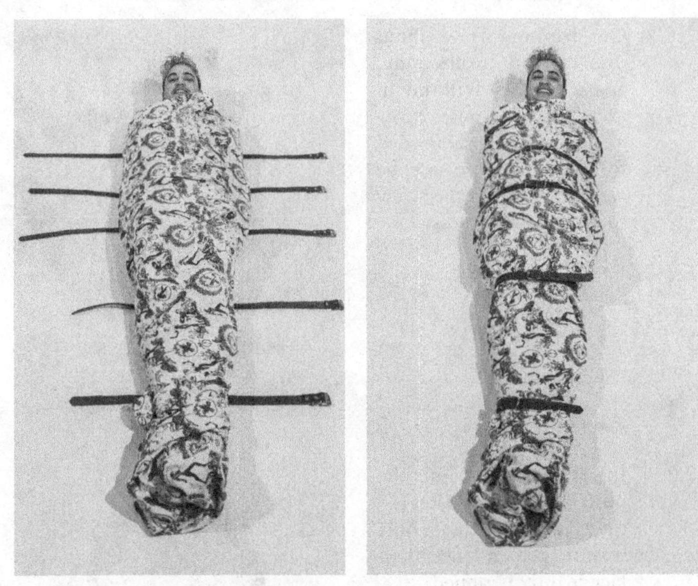

*Bottom: Gage. Top: Mildred S. Pierce.*

**Safety precautions:** Make sure not to cut off circulation by cinching the belts too tightly.

## 2. Bondage tape hood with nose tubes

2.1 Cut drinking straws about one to two inches long, and see if they will stay in your partner's nose without help. If help is needed for fit, duct tape can be wrapped around the straw to increase thickness.

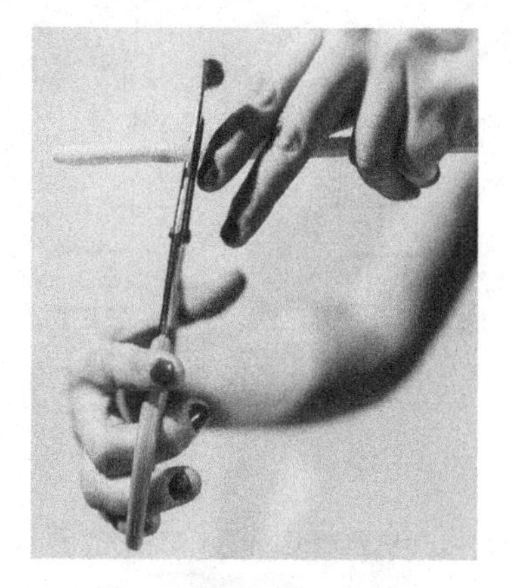

2.2 Insert the straws into the nostrils of your partner—these will be their only way to get air once their face is fully wrapped.

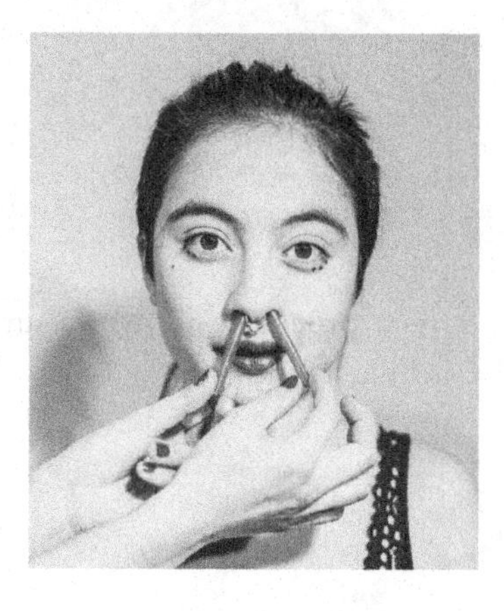

**Safety precautions:** As with all activities where the bottom is unable to speak, make sure that you have a nonverbal safeword system set up so that your partner can communicate their needs to you.

2.3 Begin wrapping the bondage tape from the crown of the head, passing the wrap underneath the chin.

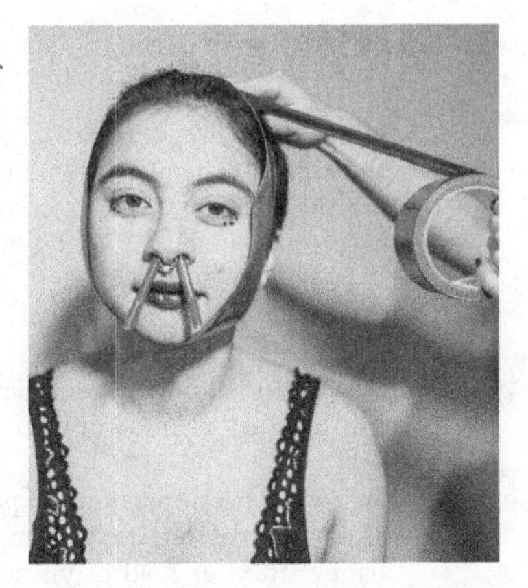

2.4 Fold the wrap and change directions, wrapping horizontally around the face, from the forehead down to the chin.

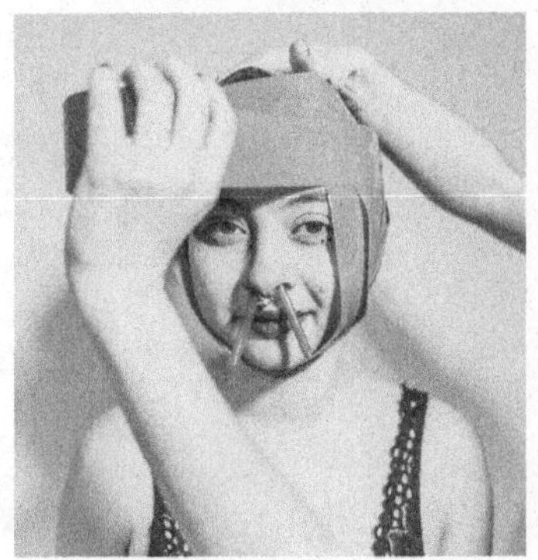

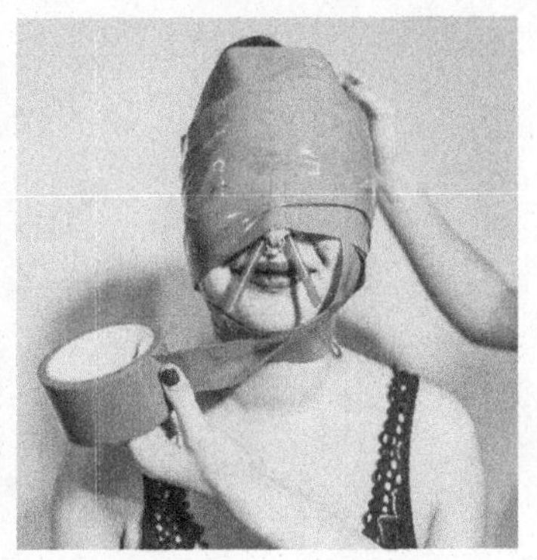

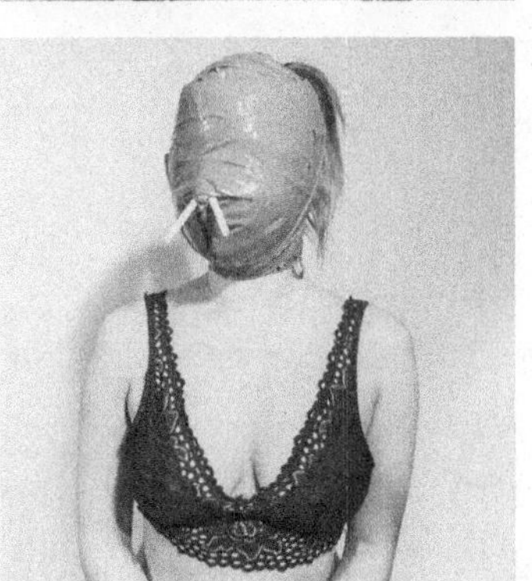

2.5 To release, simply unwrap!

*Bottom: Slice. Top: Mildred S. Pierce.*

## 3. Ganzfeld goggles

3.1 By covering a regular pair of goggles with either black or white duct tape, you can hack a pair of Ganzfeld goggles! Just make sure that the field of vision is completely one shade/color, and that there are no cracks of light getting in.

3.2 The results will vary from person to person, but the best way to get a result is to sit in a place with concentrated light, wear the goggles, and "look" or point your head toward the wall. This will ensure the most uniform light source.

3.3 Keep your eyes open and be patient! Anywhere from five to ten minutes into your wearing experience, you might begin to see changes in your field of vision, from subtle things like shadows that aren't really there to colorful, full-fledged hallucinations.

CHAPTER

11

# PHYSICALLY STRESSFUL BONDAGE

For the masochists and escape-artist types known in the bondage world as eels, physically stressful bondage is the Holy Grail of bondage activities. The intensity of the vulnerability and inescapability that are invoked through physical stress are unparalleled by other bondage activities. As we have learned, these two rewards can be highly motivating, so pushing the boundaries of bondage exploration into this realm is simply a natural progression of human curiosity. The rewards do, however, come with a steep price; physically stressful bondage is an incredibly risky and dangerous form of bondage and should only be undertaken by experienced bondage practitioners. This chapter will discuss the different types of physically stressful bondage: floorwork, suspension, and predicament bondage. Tutorials will be included for basic floorwork ties and predicaments, but not for suspension techniques, as they are best learned in a live setting with an experienced instructor.

Rope is the tool of choice for physically stressful bondage due to its roots in Japanese rope torture. As you might remember from Chapter 2, I find the transition of physically stressful bondage from a form of nonconsensual torture to an art form that values consent, safety, and comfort to be highly poetic. The shift demonstrates our ability to use consensual bondage activities to liberate and empower each other. Within that context, there is room for all sorts of bondage practitioners, as long as they are engaging with consenting partners. There are many traditionalists who still rig for pain and torture because that's what they and their partners are seeking, but there are also newer riggers, like Gorgone, who study yoga and apply concepts about anatomy and the path of least resistance to their bondage practices. While still fairly rigorous and painful, these new methods of rigging also promote wellness and comfort for the bottoms so that they can enjoy their bondage experiences for longer durations and with less wear and tear on the body. They also highlight the beauty of the human form and the amazing power and strength that it possesses.

## Floorwork

The most basic form of physically stressful bondage is floorwork that involves tying traditional Japanese rope harnesses and restraint patterns. Those who study this form of rope bondage spend hours practicing basic patterns (such as the ones from Chapter 3), working on memory, precision, and speed. Once these patterns are mastered, practitioners learn how to connect them, bending their subject into an incredibly sexy and helpless pretzel. Two highly effective traditional Japanese stress ties are the ebi/agura and reverse-ebi patterns.

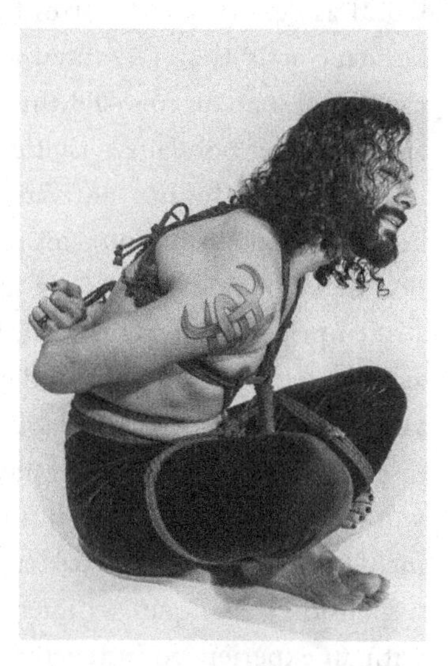

*Bottom: Hum. Top: Oz.*

**Ebi (shrimp tie):** Similar to the yogic "cat" position, the ebi—or shrimp—tie forces the bottom's body to curl forward like a shrimp, pressing the upper body close to the feet. The agura is a cross-legged variation on the torture tie, which is considerably more comfortable due to its ability to be adjusted. Most people cannot endure a completely bent position for very long before becoming drenched in sweat and overcome by back pain. Kinbaku masters who wanted to prolong the suffering of their bottoms without creating lasting damage created the agura tie as a way to improve the functionality of the traditional torture tie while maintaining its integrity. Both versions of the tie are incredibly demanding, more so than with run-of-the-mill erotic bondage, the subject should be frequently checked for proper breathing, numbness, and overall comfort.

**Reverse ebi:** Similar to the yogic "cow" position, the reverse-ebi tie curls the rope bottom backward into a bowed shape. Aesthetically it is very similar to Western hogties, where the subject's hands and feet are tied together behind the back. The main difference between the two ties is where the feet are anchored. As the reverse ebi secures the feet to a chest harness rather than to the hands, it is far more restrictive. It's also more structurally sound and is often used for horizontal suspensions.

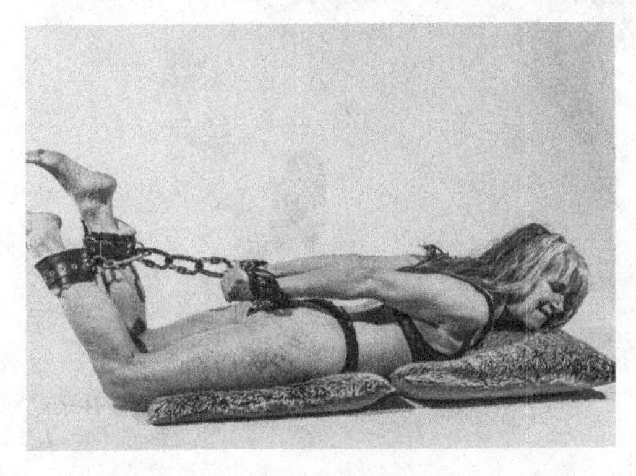

*Bottom: Simone.*
*Top: Oz.*

## Partial vs. Full Suspension

Partial suspensions build upon floorwork by supporting some of the weight of the body with bondage support lines or suspension points that connect to the basic harnesses. In partial suspension, it is common for one or two body parts to be restrained so that they cannot touch the ground, while the other limbs are left free for support. The sensation of suspension is a unique one, in that it simultaneously feels like weightlessness and heaviness. When suspended, the entire weight of the body is concentrated where the bondage devices are, and the pain of that makes you completely aware of weight. The more active a suspension bottom can be in pushing back against their restraints, the more they can support themselves rather than hanging as dead weight. This is easier to learn with "training wheels," or limbs left on the ground for weight support, hence using partial suspension as a stepping-stone to the full one.

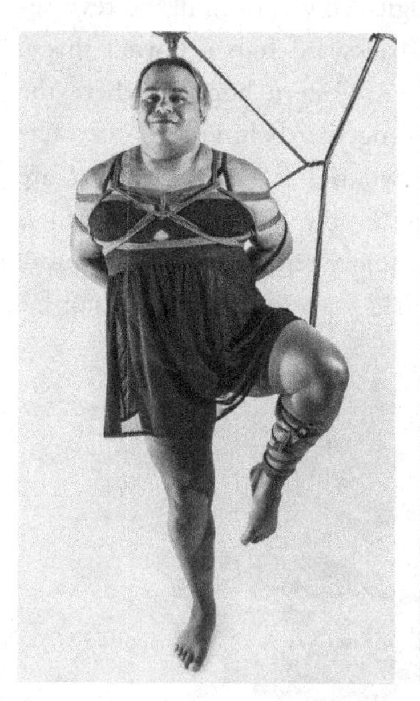

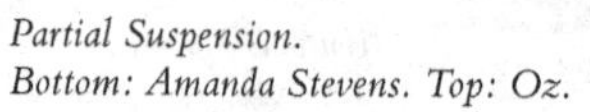

*Partial Suspension.*
*Bottom: Amanda Stevens. Top: Oz.*

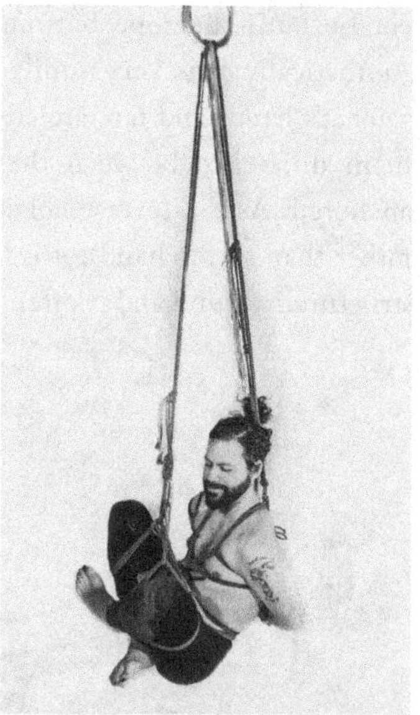

*Full Suspension. Bottom:*
*Hum. Top: Oz.*

Full suspensions involve lifting the entire body off the ground. While it is tempting to jump into full-body suspension, it is advisable to try partial suspension first to let both the bottom and the Top adjust to how the body reacts to the sensation that the bondage creates.

There are three physical orientations that are the building blocks of suspensions: horizontal, vertical, and inverted.

**Horizontal suspension:** Horizontal ties are considered to be the safest and most comfortable, as the weight can be equally distributed along the body. Beginner versions of the horizontal tie feel very similar to lying in a hammock, or swinging on a swing set with the seat balanced under your hips. In fact, if you don't want to use rope, either of those tools would be great for creating a similar sensation. Horizontal ties can be experienced either faceup or facedown, with the limbs extended for comfort or bent into a reverse ebi or other positions to increase the pain factor.

**Vertical suspension:** In the fantasyland of movies and television shows, we often see people hanging from the ceiling by their wrists. In reality, hanging from the wrists like this is incredibly dangerous and can really only be safely pulled off using special suspension cuffs that distribute the weight properly. An alternative method of vertical suspension is to use a rope harness around the waist or chest. Both of these types of harnesses come with their own set of risks, but if learned and executed properly, they can produce some incredibly stunning visuals and physical sensations.

**Inverted suspension:** Inverted suspensions can be performed using the same harnesses as vertical suspension. This creates the uniquely delightful possibility for dynamic shifts during the course of a suspension. Simply by shifting the distribution of weight, the subject can flip from right side up to upside down, or vice versa, in a matter of seconds. The ankles can also be used as a suspension point in inverted suspensions, as they're much more accustomed to bearing weight than the wrists. There is nothing quite like the sensation of being hung by the ankles! Being suspended upside down causes the blood to rush to the head and is therefore very difficult to maintain for long periods of time. Too much time upside down can cause someone to pass out, so careful communication in this type of scenario is imperative.

Why do people enjoy suspension? There are many answers to that question. Some people enjoy the artistry, while others enjoy the physical challenge. Most people enjoy it because, if done correctly, it is really fun! If approached with knowledge of the risks involved, and how to mitigate them effectively, suspension bondage with the right partner(s) can be a thrill! Look at some of the amazing things that riggers Oz and Cassivini were able to do with the help of their rope bottoms Duchess Jealoquin, Hum, and Quest! Don't be fooled. Even though the models look graceful and comfortable, they're actively participating in holding their own weight. Hum and Quest were quite sore the next day, even though they both stretched. We all think it was worth it.

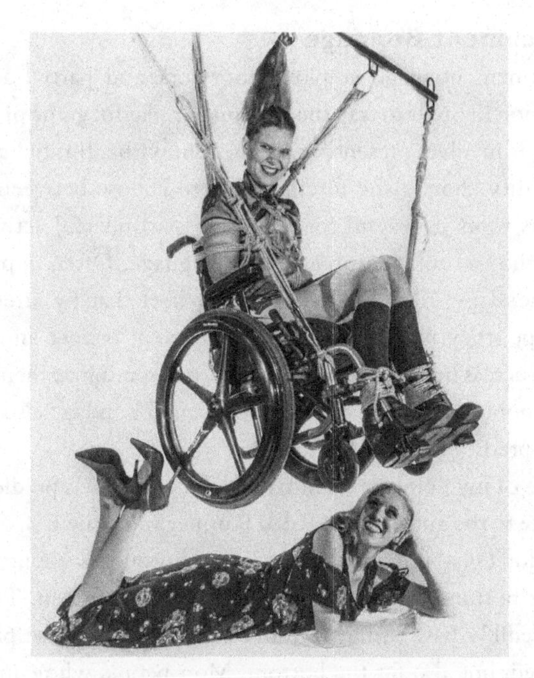

*Bottom: Duchess Jealoquin. Tops: Cassivini and Oz.*
*Model: Mistress Couple.*

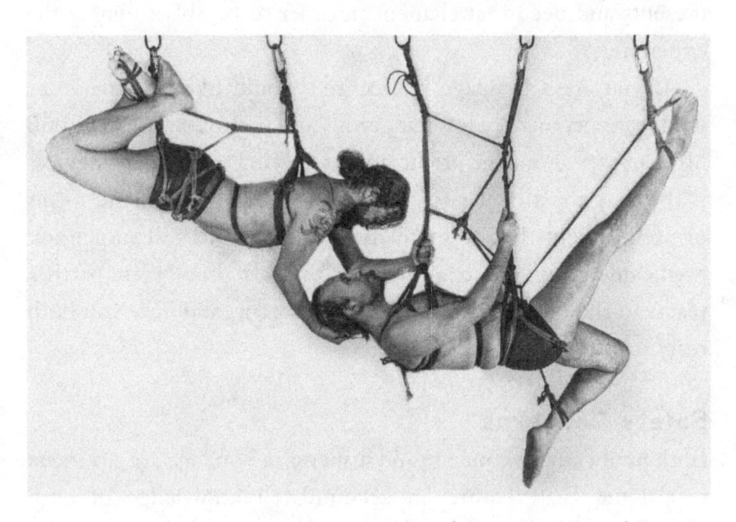

*Bottoms: Hum and Quest. Tops: Oz and Cassivini.*

## Predicament Bondage

Predicament bondage employs floorwork and partial and full suspension in order to trap the bottom in a playful game of cat and mouse. It involves presenting the bottom with a limited number of mobility choices and forcing them to choose between them. With its roots in playful torment, it is a wonderful activity for those who use antagonism as a love language. Often in predicament bondage, the subject is made to feel that by attempting to escape, they may increase their suffering, trigger an adverse effect (such as being doused by water), or even injure themselves. In this light, a significant amount of mental bondage also plays a part in predicament bondage.

One of my bondage mentors humorously likens predicament bondage to the antics of the Road Runner and Wile E. Coyote—if you don't plan out your predicament thoroughly enough, your devious bottom will be able to thwart your evil plan. This can be incredibly frustrating not only for the Top, whose plan has backfired, but also for the bottom. Most people who consent to predicament bondage really enjoy the mental challenge that it presents and need that element in order to be able to enjoy the experience.

If you are a bondage novice and would like to experience predicaments that are less dangerous and require less skill to pull off than rope-bondage predicaments, relying on bondage devices is the way to go (refer to Chapter 4). Performing basic forms of predicaments before graduating to partial or full suspension predicaments will also allow you to learn how your partner reacts to the physical stress of a predicament, and how you both react to stress under pressure.

## Safety Concerns

Both predicament bondage and suspension bondage are advanced techniques that require an accumulated knowledge of both topping and bottoming skills. Due to the variety of potentially hazardous challenges that physically stressful bondage presents, the bottom must take a more active role than usual in supporting their weight against the restraints, and also in speaking up about discomfort. It is likely that the suffering involved in a physically stressful bondage position allows the bottoms to drop into their bodies and focus on their physical states rather than the world around them. Their attention turns from the outward stressors of everyday life to the physical stress they are experiencing in the moment. As the director of this physically and mentally demanding experience, the Top must stay vigilant. Similar to when playing chess, a bondage Top needs to be thinking five steps ahead. Things for the Top to consider include the safety and comfort of the bottom, how to transition them in and out of positions, what kind of mental landscape these positions are going to create for the bottom, and the mechanics of the bondage devices. Physically stressful bondage is no walk in the park, and it should be clear to you why learning these skills thoroughly takes a great deal of time.

## TUTORIALS

### 1. Predicament Tutorial

1.1 Attach suspension cuffs to secure hard points in the ceiling.
1.2 Have your bottom stand on their toes.
1.3 Place something uncomfortable under their feet (rice, rocks, acupressure mat, tea light candles).
1.4 Your submissive now has the option of holding themselves up with the cuffs or relaxing their arms and letting their weight fall on whatever is under their feet. The choice is to either put strain on the shoulders or cause pain under the feet.

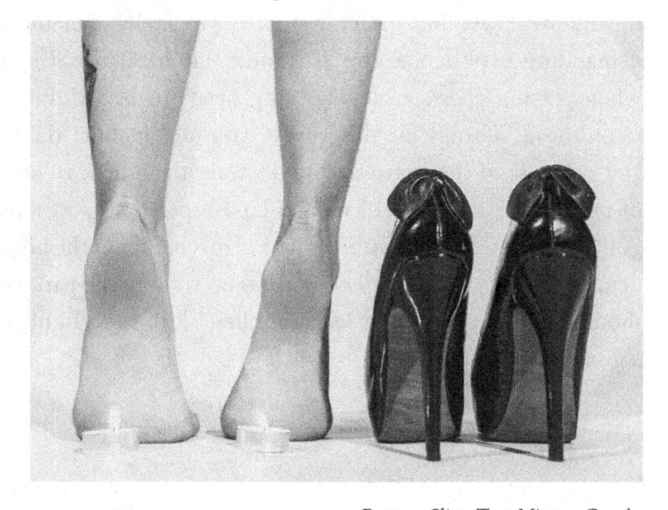

*Bottom: Slice. Top: Mistress Couple.*

CHAPTER

12

# SELF-BONDAGE

Unfortunately, we're coming to the final destination of our bondage journey. Now that you have an in-depth knowledge of the gamut of bondage activities that exist, why not try some out on yourself? Self-bondage is one of the best ways to learn about how different types of bondage affect you. After all, you have the best understanding out of anyone of what your interests and limits are, what speed to proceed at, and how far to push. Similar to masturbation, self-bondage allows you to explore your own body and figure out what you like/dislike before inviting others into the equation. This chapter will highlight how applying bondage to yourself is the most dangerous form of bondage that you can engage in. We will discuss some methods of risk reduction, which devices are best for safer self-bondage practices, and even learn how to create your own safer self-bondage devices out of household items. Then, you'll be left to your own devices to practice all of the knowledge that you've accumulated in the course of reading this book!

## Motivations for Engaging in Self-Bondage

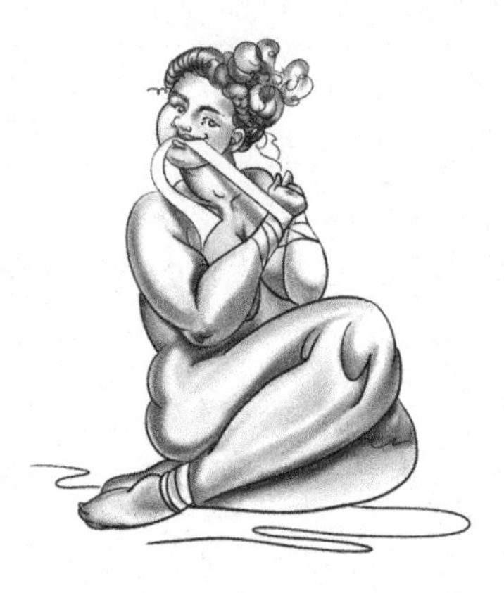

Many folks choose to engage in self-bondage as a self-care exercise, very much like a yoga practice or meditation. For others, it is purely a sexual endeavor. Whatever the motivation is, solo bondage produces the unique dichotomy of making you both captor and captive. Being in control of your own captivity comes with its own distinct set of pros and cons, most of which come down to the concept of self-preservation. For instance, the benefit of agency over your body comes with the drawback that there is no spotter and therefore an increased amount of risk involved with doing bondage alone. Self-bondage is comparable to tying someone else up and leaving them alone—the risk of any accident, from a house fire to a heart attack, may be extremely slight, but when you're helplessly bound and left alone, there's little to no margin of safety. Along the same lines, no matter how sadistic a bondage partner might be, they will most likely intend to set you free at some point, and if they're a good partner, they'll take precautions to ensure that your limits are respected until that happens. With self-bondage, you're on your own; one accidental slipup and you could end up seriously hurt, or even dead. For that reason, it is my strong recommendation that self-bondage be practiced in the presence of another person or with another person nearby.

For those who crave the sensations of immobility and restraint regardless of how easy the bonds are to escape, sensual self-bondage is the approach to explore. Practicing the activities in this book with a pair of safety shears or set of keys nearby will not make it any less enjoyable; in fact, knowing that you have a way out in case of emergency might make it more fun. Wearing the body harness from Chapter 7 while you do chores around your house or practicing the futomomo on your own legs will allow you to experience and appreciate the activities on your own terms.

For those who crave the sensation of helplessness and do not have the option to be restrained by a partner, strict self-bondage is the only answer. In strict self-bondage, the goal is to recreate the experience of being under the control of a Top, and to make it feel as real as possible.[92] These types of predicaments are incredibly difficult, if not impossible, to escape without the implementation of some sort of self-timed or punishment-based mechanism to release the bondage. The helplessness created by this type of scenario is even more intense than being restrained by a capable partner. If the restraint becomes uncomfortable, painful, or even dangerous, there is no one to release you, no safeword system in place. Despite the risk involved with this type of bondage, many strict self-bondage practitioners are thrill seekers and feel that "if you can let yourself out at any time, why bother do it at all?"[93]

---

92 David Stein, "Doing It Yourself," *AltSex* (blog), 1995, https://web.archive.org/web/20021202101120/http://www.altsex.org/bdsm/self-bd-1.html.

93 Ibid.

## Materials for Self-Bondage

### *Self-Timed Release Systems*

Self-timed restraints allow you to escape restraints after a predetermined period of time. Some are more reliable than others, so it is advisable to get well acquainted with the device before using it on yourself. After all, this device is acting as your spotter, partner, and ultimately your captor and rescuer, so you're going to want to know it intimately before trusting it with your life. Setting up a self-bondage predicament can be incredibly challenging. Even the simplest setups require a lot of planning. For instance, if you're using handcuffs and locks, pinning the keys on the ledge of the table, underneath your phone, is a good example of a self-timed release system. In this scenario, it is important to use the keys to open the lock before doing anything else. Then set the timer to vibrate the phone after a specific duration of time, and learn to place the keys just so that when the phone vibrates, the keys are dropped to the floor. Open the lock, position yourself, apply the cuffs, and then lock them together. You won't need the keys for this if the lock is already opened. Then, you can lie on the floor restrained until the keys fall and you're able to grab them to release your bonds. Because of the elaborate nature of these escape mechanisms, it is really important to practice and master them before getting yourself into a dangerous predicament!

If you're feeling adventurous, other self-timed release systems include:

- Ice and ice locks: Though a bit fickle to control, ice and ice locks are some of the most commonly utilized self-timed release devices. A key can be placed in water, which is then frozen, only becoming available for use once the ice melts. Ice locks are frozen together and do not release until the ice has melted. Though it can be difficult to gauge precisely how long the scenario will last using ice, it is simple to use and reliable that it will melt eventually, as long as the room is set at a fairly warm temperature.
- Combination locks: Resetting combination locks can be useful, as they rely on the time needed to try every possibility for an unknown combination. Do not use the kind of combination lock that you used on your locker in high school, with numbers going up to forty and endless permutations. Instead use combination padlocks that are limited to three or four single-digit dials. Typically, it takes fifteen to twenty minutes to solve a three-digit combination lock, and about two hours to crack a four-digit lock, accounting for less time if the combination starts with lower numbers, and more time if it starts with higher numbers. Combination locks can also be used in the dark of night, only able to be solved once the light of morning reveals the combination dial.

A word of warning regarding ice locks, based on Master R's first experience with one:

"Mistakes are made. Ice locks make great self-bondage tools, but . . . I had tied myself pretty thoroughly with my hands attached to the ice lock directly above my head. I also had my legs in a spreader bar and my cock filled with an electrified urethral plug. I would be in that position until the ice lock thawed. I could barely move with all the counterbalances I had incorporated in my tie. That's when it happened. I suddenly had a drop of water land on the top of my head. Then another, and then another . . . The ice lock was melting directly above me, and the water was dripping, one rhythmic, slow, Chinese-water-torture drop at a time, directly on the very top of my head. It was truly maddening. It went for about twenty minutes. I attempted to twist and turn my way into avoidance. Toward the end, while bending my back in the most awkward way, I managed to get myself stuck in a slightly altered position. The water no longer fell on my head. Instead, going straight down, it was now falling directly on my tied cock—which, if you recall, had an electrified sound in it. I spent the next terrifying five minutes waiting for the worst. After five minutes, thank the goddess, the ice lock was empty. I was wet and horrified over what the outcome could have been. Yes, ice locks are a means of escapable self-bondage, but still, it is always advisable in life to have a backup plan."

### *Punishment-Based Release Systems*

A compromise between safety and strictness involves the use of a punishment-based release system, or booby trap. These devices allow you to escape immediately, but only at the cost of some penalty with their use. For example, keys could be placed in a bucket of oil or paint to discourage their use. In the case of an emergency, the safety of release would outweigh the detriment of having to clean up the mess, but otherwise you would remain bound until the predetermined duration was reached. Other examples of punishment-based release systems include storing the key at the bottom of a container with unpleasant (not poisonous!) food or drink that must be consumed in order to get to the key, or the terrifying prospect of having to call someone for help.

## TUTORIALS

### 1. How to Make an Ice Lock

Note: This tutorial assumes a basic understanding of how to safely use the materials and tools listed below. If you are not comfortable using these materials or tools safely, we suggest enlisting the assistance of someone proficient in the techniques described below. Please also note that this tutorial requires a safe workspace for using a power drill. Improper use of power tools may result in injury.

#### *Materials:*

★ All metal parts are stainless steel.

1 - 1"x1½" PVC reducer

1 - 1"x1½" PVC end cap

1 - 1" rubber stopper

1 - ¼"x3" eye bolt (Each eye bolt should come with a ¼"-20 tpi nut. If it does not, purchase one)

1 - ¼"x2" eye bolt (Each eye bolt should come with a ¼"-20 tpi nut. If it does not, purchase one)

2 - ¼"x1" flat metal washers (Ask the hardware store for a fender washer)

1 - ¼"x1" rubber washer

#### *Tools:*

1 - drill

1 - ¼" drill bit

1 - pair of pliers

1.1 Start by drilling a quarter-inch hole through the one-inch rubber stopper.

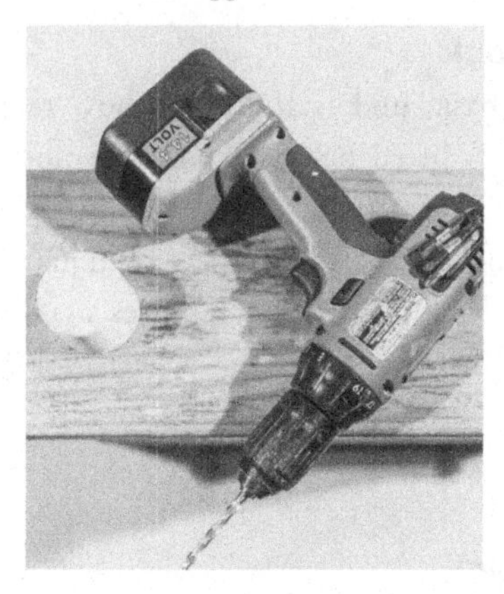


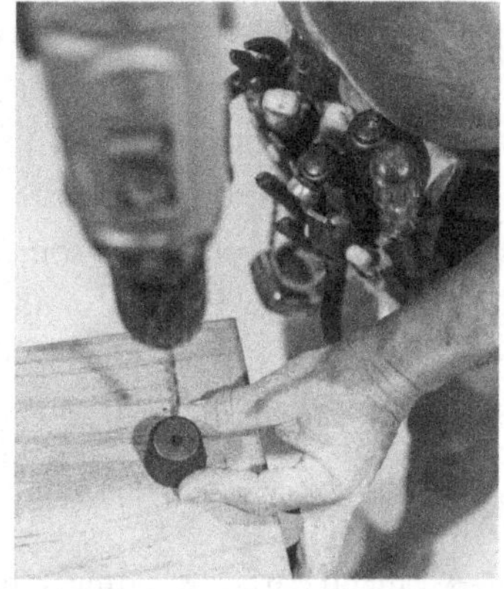

1.2 Insert the ¼"x3" eye bolt through the hole in the stopper, so that the eye of the bolt is protruding from the wider end of the stopper.

1.3 Slip the ¼"x1" fender washer on the end of the eye bolt, followed by one of the ¼"-20 nuts, and tighten to the bottom of the stopper.

1.4 Next drill a quarter-inch hole in the center of the PVC end cap.

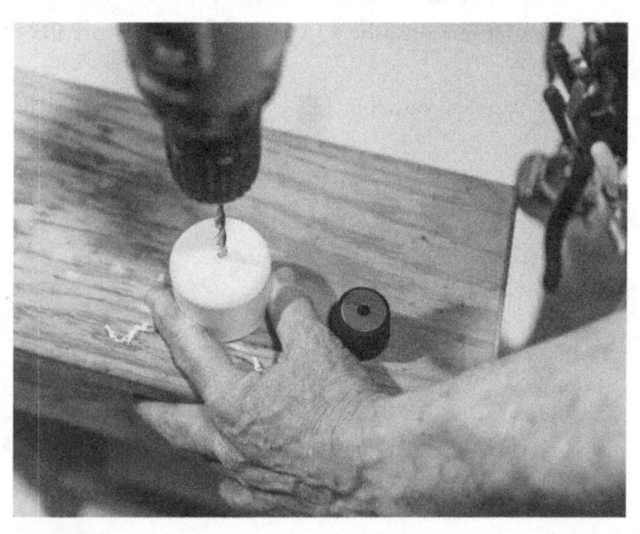

1.5 Insert the ¼"x2" eye bolt through the drilled hole in the end cap, so that the eye of the bolt is protruding from the closed end of the cap.

1.6 Slip the ¼"x1" rubber washer on the end of the eye bolt, followed by the other ¼"x1" fender washer, and finally a ¼"-20 nut. Tighten with pliers to compress the rubber washer.

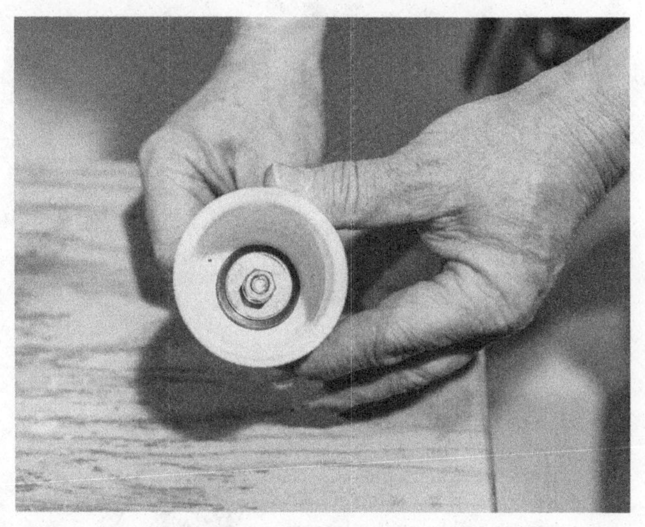

1.7 Fit the 1"x1½" PVC reducer into the end cap and squeeze them together to create the housing for the ice lock. At this point, the assembly should look like a teacup with an eye bolt coming out of the bottom.

1.8 Fill the ice lock housing that you have created with water, just as you would fill a teacup.

1.9 Insert the stopper assembly in the open end of the PVC reducer, to create a light watertight seal. There is no need to jam the stopper in as if you were corking a bottle of wine—in fact, if you do this, you might cause the device to fail. The rubber stopper is simply meant to hold the water inside the lock. Once stopped, freeze the full ice lock anywhere from thirty minutes to overnight depending on how strong you want the lock to be. The longer you freeze the lock, the longer it will take to defrost.

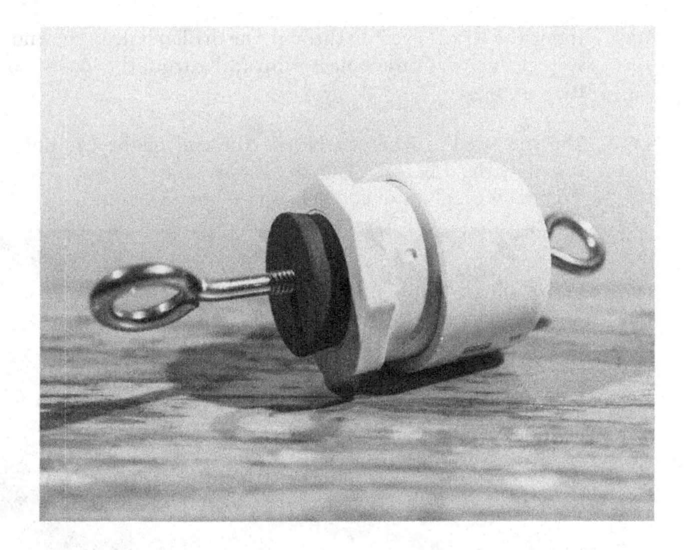

1.10 Be sure to test the release time by hanging a five-pound weight from the lock and observing how long it takes to release. Once the ice has melted, the rubber stopper assembly will separate from the ice-lock housing, simultaneously releasing the mechanism and freeing the prisoner. It might take a few trials to perfect the release mechanism.

1.11 Once you have established the release time, you can freeze the lock again and use it to anchor yourself to a piece of furniture or lock your limbs together. The bondage will remain effective until the ice melts and releases the lock mechanism.

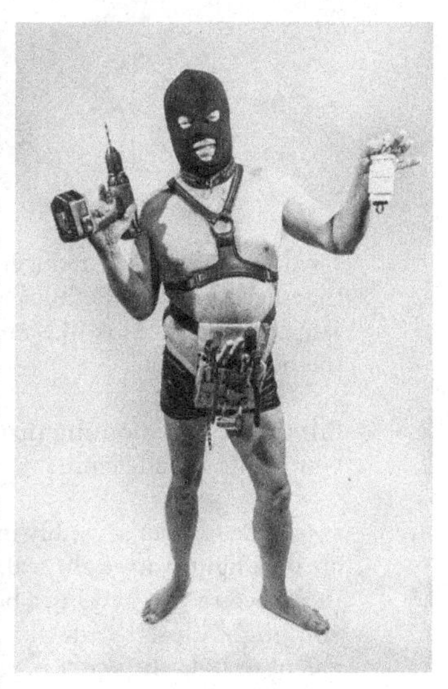

*Top and Bottom: slave 9.*

### Instructions on Freeze Time

Other factors that determine freeze time include the amount of water used in the lock, elevation, room temperature, and body temperature, so be prepared to account for those differences.

SECTION 3:

# EROTIC ESSAYS

Now that you know all about the ten realms of bondage and have tried some of the tutorials, you might be wondering how to construct a bondage scene to play out with your partner. Scene construction could take an entire separate book to explain, so I've tried to help you by taking a different route. In the following pages, you will read essays written by me and my friends, partners, and bondage bottoms. Each of these essays was written with a prompt associated with one of the ten realms of bondage that you learned about in Section 2, and aims to create the landscape for you to insert yourself into the scene. Each essay will talk about the writer's physical, mental, and emotional experiences while engaging in bondage activities. It is my hope that by reading these examples of bondage scenes and scenarios, you will be able to start imagining some sexy bondage scenarios of your own! As you will see, some of these essays include multiple types of bondage, because in reality BDSM scenes are never as cut-and-dried as a book chapter! You should feel free to mix and match as many bondage techniques as you'd like once you venture off to play with these concepts. Enjoy!

CHAPTER

13

# JAPANESE ROPE BONDAGE

## The God Particle

***By Daemonumx***

On an otherwise normal Tuesday afternoon, I received an intriguing message from another queer femme I had met at a few kink events. She had wanted to experience rope bondage for quite some time and felt brave enough to ask me if I would tie her up. Her message was written with deliberate words and gracious prose showing definite signs of submission.

I assigned her an essay that asked her to answer a few questions: "What kind of experience would you like to have?" and "What is your relationship to pain?" She sent me photos of a two-page handwritten letter in which she described intimately her desire to be bound and used to my liking, to submit to my fierce femininity. "I'll love being immobilized and reanimated by you when you tie me . . . I have a dark fantasy of being turned into the God particle." Scientists believe that the God particle is what sparked creation, turning mass into matter. Her fantasy was to feel grounded in her body with rope bondage as the vehicle for this transformation.

*She gets it*, I thought. Never had I been approached so genuinely with such vulnerability. It ignited my Top creativity. I was drawn to her ideas, and I began to fantasize about the ways I would torture her. One thing was clear—she wanted a journey back home to her body after a lifetime of trauma made it all too easy to dissociate.

The pain and suffering of rope suspension has the unique ability to both immediately ground and liberate someone. Imagine your body tightly constricting and contorting to another's complete desire, while your mind feels freer than ever before. To withstand the pain, you must focus on your breath and settle into each position, homing in on every compression, every torsion. Your mind, however, is free to depart.

She came to my house a few days later. After much careful discussion around pain and the ways it helps us move through trauma, we began the session. Her undressing revealed an emerald-green silk lingerie set framed with lace. "I went shopping today for the occasion; I bought this just for you," she announced proudly.

"On your knees," I told her, not wasting any time and refusing to be distracted. I knelt behind her and brought her arms behind her back. I began by tying a TK (Takate-Kote) chest harness that squeezed her incredible breasts tightly together. Next, I pulled her off her knees so she was sitting on the floor. I added a suspension line from the back of the chest harness up to the bamboo beam to load her weight into a partial suspension. Watching her struggle to reach the ground, I pulled her legs apart so that her ass was barely touching the floor.

"Remember that pain you asked for?" I reminded her of that plea to submit to my will as I began to clip clothespins down her inner thigh, one by one, over a scarlet piece of thread. I placed a few more on her stomach and began to play with them to see what intensity would cause her to scream out, gauging her pain threshold. She proved to be quite tough, flinching only slightly as I tapped and flicked the pins that pinched her flesh. It wasn't until I began pulling the string—slowly ripping each clothespin off—that she screamed and cursed. She was glad to accept my gift of torture.

Next, I quickly tied her right leg in a futomomo and tied a single column on her left ankle. "On to your next level of pain," I teased as I lifted her in the air, one leg after the other. Her breathing changed, becoming deeper.

"Oh my God!" she gasped. With the pain of suspension radiating, she could feel every inch of her body, something she told me she hadn't felt in so long—something that's really difficult for a lot of us who carry trauma in our flesh and bones.

The chest harness suspended from the back, combined with both legs in the air, brought her into a facedown position. Once she was settled there, I began to transition her to hanging upside down by her legs by removing the line on the chest harness. Her continued deep exhales were a sign of her pleasure in the intensity. I grabbed my scratchiest coconut rope and wrapped it once around her thigh, pulling very tight in opposite directions. She let out a beautiful scream, just as I expected, pleasing the sadist in me.

"Has anyone ever orgasmed in your ropes?" she asked.

"Why? Are you going to orgasm?" I countered.

"I think I could, if I had something on my clit," she said. She seemed like she was curious to see what might happen.

"I can fix that." Before she knew it, I had roped her into a tight chastity belt with extreme pressure on her clit. I had already brought her back to a facedown position, so gravity was on her side.

She rocked herself back and forth as I brought her legs up even higher to give her just the right amount of pressure on her pussy rope. Suddenly she started moaning in a pulsing rhythm that was music to my ears. She was making the most blissful face, on display for me, with her hair tied back to the chest line. It was a powerful experience to witness her hanging there, so vulnerable, finding the ultimate pleasure in her pain.

"Good girl," I said to her, grabbing her face. "You came for me. Very, very good girl."

With her body still shaking, mine tired and sweaty, I began to untie her hair and clit rope first for some immediate release. Then I lowered her chest and legs down, one by one, until she was curled up in a puddle on the floor with the happiest smirk I'd seen in a while.

She lay quietly for a few minutes. When she came back to earth and could articulate her thoughts, she said, "That was so healing, thank you." Her body language confirmed it, and I could feel her energy had shifted. As I untied her, I reflected on her fantasy to be turned into a God particle. In a way, that fantasy had come true: Her experience of pain brought her from floating mass to corporeal matter, sparking a deep reconnection with her body—if only for the session.

After she was untied and dressed, we spoke intimately for a while. She had used pain as a vehicle for escape for as long as she could remember. Using pain as an exercise in embodiment was a completely new, cathartic experience. Handing over trust and responsibility while immobilized is not an easy task. I told her how pleased I was that she accepted the pain and the journey; I was glad to be able to give her the experience she so badly sought.

As I walked her to the door, I leaned in to whisper, "I think you might be ready for your next assignment."

CHAPTER

# 14

# DEVICE BONDAGE

## Device of Destiny

***By slave Destiny***

"Being your slave, what should I do but tend upon the hours and times of your desire! I have no precious time at all to spend, nor service to do, till you require . . ." —William Shakespeare[94]

I am in posture, kneeling, hands open, fingers apart, offering myself for my Mistress's pleasure, waiting, quivering with anticipation. A sound—it is the door opening followed by the click of boot heels on the stairs. Every atom of my being is alive, longing to see Her, the Mistress to whom I have dedicated myself.

The curtain parts and my gaze falls upon the most beautiful woman I have ever known. She is wearing a black corset, opera-length gloves, and tall black leather boots, a sight so entrancing that I scarcely remember to breathe. The sight of Mistress Couple fills me with dreams few mortals dare to dream. Soon, soon I will be transported to another realm.

I am a slave, Her slave, and She is both my Mistress and the love of my life. She speaks and I feel both Her power and Her

---

94 Shakespeare, William. *Sonnet 57*. Ed. Amanda Mabillard. *Shakespeare Online*. 8 Dec. 2008. http://www.shakespeare-online.com/sonnets/57detail.html.

love, and for a moment She holds me close. In Her hand is a black leather posture collar inscribed with my name, Destiny. It was given to me on the day she accepted me as Her personal slave. As the collar tightens, we are bound together in mind and body, Mistress and slave.

She leads me to a large wooden cross and begins to place leather restraints around my wrists and ankles; I become helpless and vulnerable, totally in her power. How I have been longing for this moment! It is both an act of submission and an offering of love in which one party gives themself without reservation to another.

I now feel an almost electric sensation as a cord tightens around my genitals. My balls are gently stretched down toward the earth and my cock, growing engorged, becomes harder than I can fathom.

Mistress appears before me with a pair of floggers, which She softly brushes against my lust-filled bones in a lingering and sensual caress. Then She begins, the floggers crossing over each other and striking my hungry flesh. I feel the thump against my chest and then the sting, which sets my senses ablaze. Straining against the bonds securing me, I present my body to Her by pushing toward the source of the blows.

She methodically moves down my body from chest to stomach, creeping closer and closer to my immobilized genitals. In my mind, I am begging, longing for the blows to rain upon my most sensitive areas. Then, finally, the blows begin to fall upon my jutting cock, and at each strike it assumes a life of its own, becoming longer, harder, eagerly begging for more.

The boundary between pleasure and pain is now crossed, and one enhances the other in a never-ending cycle of euphoric sensory stimulation. After a momentary pause, a new implement, a whip with a single tail, brushes the head of my cock so softly, whispering against my skin. Next, it shouts, a crushing blow, as the whip wraps around my shaft, pulling at my member, which continues to vibrate as the lash retreats. Mistress's attention now focuses upon the restrained testicles, which jump and shudder with each blow of the whip. The intensity of sensation is almost overwhelming, and yet I never wish to beg for mercy because the raining blows are bringing me to a new pinnacle of pleasure. I willingly sacrifice myself to my Mistress and in return, I am showered with her love and attention.

I am called Destiny, and I am both a submissive and, more importantly, a slave who has freely offered himself to Mistress Couple, and has been accepted by Her. A distinction should be made between the two concepts of submissive and slave, the latter having a connotation that many might find reprehensible. The key is, I want to be Mistress Couple's property. I want to be owned by Her, used by Her, and I want to be as useful to Her as the tools or devices that She uses to restrain me. I have completely surrendered myself to Her, and in service to Her, the self-serving aspects of my character have been stripped away. The resulting intensity of love and devotion that I have experienced through service to Her surpasses anything I have known before.

I have attempted in these pages to describe what I have experienced, knowing that these words are woefully inadequate. They cannot explain what I feel in Her presence. Perhaps this simple metaphor will leave you with a deeper understanding of our dynamic: The connection forged between us is stronger and more enduring than the most durable devices in Her dungeon.

CHAPTER

15

# MENTAL BONDAGE

## Clarity and Devotion

***By Domina Claire Hex, with consent from John***

I've often wondered whether religion is the root of my kinks, or simply my earliest exposure to themes of power and devotion. Rituals for worship, suffering for transcendence, and the concept of belonging to something absolute . . . For me, the leap to bondage wasn't far.

For John, an attraction to bondage preceded religion. Religion was the remedy to the shame of his kinks. He became an ordained minister, vowing to root out his submissive nature and live obediently under God. This stage in John's life was temporary, and when he broke from the church, he emerged with a renewed desire to make his fem-dom dreams a reality.

I was not John's first Domme, nor was he my first sub, but the dedication that sparked between us was unprecedented. Together we flipped our shared background on its head, defining what we held as sacred, and ritualizing a celebration of female power. I beat him with all my strength and the utmost care. In the heat and the long afterglow, I could practically levitate.

Although we lived in different states and in-person meetings were a treat, John soon became my 24/7 devoted disciple.

"You have truly become my Goddess and Religion," he wrote. I reveled in the embodiment of sacred humanity, sacred everything. I knew that John's surrender was a gift, and also that I must be thoughtful with the Dominant power I possessed. Role play is one thing. Religion is another.

We started with prayers, to be memorized and recited daily. We had a prayer for meals, dedicating to myself a meditation on the sensory experience of eating, and thanking all "The worms and plants and animals/Including the humans who labored" to produce John's food. Another prayer for confession. Another prayer to me, dedicating his service to my power ("Your presence is divine"), outlining basic ethics ("For you I will do my best/To affect the world in a way/That will not cause harm to others/or myself"), and establishing the basis of our exchange ("I am yours because I want to be/And because you grant me the privilege").

The significance of this particular verse of mine had always been a theological sticking point for John—free will versus determinism. "Being My slave is something you must choose for yourself," I wrote. "Not just once, but every day. Likewise, being your Owner is My choice." I explained that my power was built out of layers of free will. His will to submit, my will to dominate. John would have preferred a more "inescapable" bondage model, with his own free will washed down the drain. To me, it was imperative, and only realistic, to keep his underlying agency intact.

I immersed myself in books on the Divine Feminine, transcendental uses of pain, and the role of ritual in organized belief. I issued regular journal assignments. The journals were a supplemental outlet for John, an exercise for his mind and a window into it. I tasked him to write about his fantasies, his past, and his daily routines.

Reading through John's Daily Routines report, I highlighted the most fertile areas—existing routines that could easily be modified into meaningful ritual and service. Also notable were areas in which John could clearly be happier and healthier. Where John might not possess the motivation to improve his life for his own sake, he held a great deal of potential, and I knew that I could motivate him to clear certain obstacles.

On Sundays, John was forbidden to eat meat, in line with his owner's ethics. This was a rule he broke once, succumbing to lobster at a seafood restaurant. His punishment was to spend fifteen minutes filming a live lobster tank in public, and to send me the recording. I wanted him to meditate on the difference between consensual bondage and the real torture these animals endured. Thoroughly humiliated by the task, and horrified by what he saw, John never broke this commandment again.

Mental training at a distance fueled physical training in person. Flogging, whipping, electric shock. My spit in his eye. I left him with a face slap and a hug.

As a symbol of my ownership, John wore a locking ankle bracelet, kept hidden under his sock, while I wore the key. He desperately wanted a locking day collar, too, one that could pass in public. We scoured the internet for an innocuous design, finally settling on a subtle combination-lock necklace. Only I knew the combo, and locking it in place gave me immense satisfaction . . . but saying goodbye that day, I felt a twinge of anxiety. What if the necklace caught on something, and my disciple strangled himself? Though I recognized the scenario as unlikely, it was difficult to sleep that week. I commanded John to come into the city, with minimal explanation. I needed to remove that collar.

"Goddess," John said when he arrived, "my day collar has been falling off."

We replaced the faulty collar with a necklace pendant. On one side, Clarity. On the other, Devotion.

As one year passed, and we became closer, it became clear to me that John was missing fulfillment in other areas of his life. He hated his job. I commanded him to research alternatives. He lacked a significant outlet for his creative talent. I commanded him to write short stories. He was lonely and isolated. I commanded him to attend his first munch.

Meanwhile, my attention was becoming more divided. To maintain a healthy stable of multiple submissives is no easy task, when you are a goddess but still only human. I struggled to give John the attention he desired, and to maintain the level of communication he had come to expect. I gave him a package of seeds, as an assignment. He was to plant and care for them and document their growth for me.

On New Year's Day, I received a surprising email from Disciple John. He wanted me to set him free.

Could he, he asked, continue to see me, while also worshipping beauty in nature and other forms? Could he see other Dommes if he wanted, and even try dating? He wanted to get his career on track, to channel his free will and creativity into other interests and talents. "Please have mercy, and be gracious to me."

I was stunned and grinning, overflowing with happiness for my disciple, amazed at his self-determination. I could not have imagined a more positive evolution for both of us, though I never expected him to initiate the parting. John's uncollaring ceremony was celebratory and steeped in ritual—candles, oils, invocations, and rites of pain. We emerged from the dungeon feeling very light and free, and are each living zealously today.

CHAPTER 16

# OBJECTIFICATION BONDAGE

## Toy

### *By Domina Franco*

Todd and Elise had been so comfortable with each other in those first weeks of dating that conversations about BDSM and the intricacies of their desires and limits were completely natural. Both had been frustrated, historically pigeonholed into primarily vanilla or Dominant roles with the partners they had before meeting each other. He was a tall, meaty man with thighs like tree trunks. He was Ivy League educated and worked on Wall Street. She was just a few inches shorter than him, a curvy Amazon with wide shoulders, pale, creamy skin, and thick, dark hair. She had often joked that her time spent working as a Dominatrix had made her an amazing negotiator and influencer, helping her immensely in her career as a marketing manager at a PR firm. Somehow they had found each other, both switches fluctuating beautifully between Dominant and submissive tendencies in equal measure.

Todd's desire to submit, which had been stifled for so long, broke the dam, the rush of wanting to be used clearing away everything that had been before. Seeing the shift in Todd and guiding the power exchange was intoxicating for Elise.

She would often be in the middle of a client presentation the morning following one of their dates with the delicious distraction of her thumping clit as she tried to focus. She wondered if people could smell her. She knew her panties were wet. Could her clients sense who she was outside this conference room? She oscillated between wanting to ensure her sex life remained a secret and being excited that people might feel it rippling off her as she sauntered down the sidewalks of New York, waited in line for coffee, or bought raspberries at the market.

One evening Todd sheepishly asked to strip off all his clothes and lie at her feet. He liked the idea of lying on the floor with her feet covering his face, switching off his brain as she did her nails and watched her favorite TV shows. How lovely it was to feel her heels resting on his eye sockets, the high arches of her feet making a bridge over the crest of his nose and her toes sitting gently on the cushions of his warm lips. Watching his cock get hard as she filed her nails and silently applied her polish made her heart swell. As their relationship progressed, he would hold her legs up while they fucked and firmly press her feet to his face. While he couldn't see, Elise would watch his body moving like an animal as he slid inside her. He had quickly evolved into a very enthusiastic and joyfully compliant toy. There were many ways Todd served Elise, but this was by far her favorite. She loved making him nothing but a vehicle for her pleasure and teasing him by describing all the ways she planned on using him. She would whisper into his ear about making him crawl across the floor in a room full of Dommes, serving each one of them as an oral slave until they had all been satisfied. She loved watching him react as she made new degrading pet names for him. They would cuddle afterward, peppering each other with gentle kisses while smiles spread over their faces. It surprised Elise. This was love.

The relationship progressed as relationships do. The incremental days strung into weeks, and into months. Each moment built something deeper than the sweat and sex. There was an uncomfortably cold but romantic ride on the Wonder Wheel at Coney Island, countless dinner dates, visits to the city's museums and walks through Central Park. She told him more about her time as a Domme and about her experience with submissive men. She described a friend's dungeon outside the city as one of the most erotic, emotionally transformative, and well-stocked spaces she had ever played. It wasn't long afterward that they were headed outside New York to this private place in the woods. The road stretched ahead, and they laughed that some couples go apple picking in the fall but they preferred to go to a basement full of chastity devices, nipple clamps, and floggers.

Sonja's cabin was quaint and homey. The small wood-burning stove on a brick hearth cranked out incredible heat, which felt wonderful as they came inside from the crisp afternoon. It was best to keep Sonja's slaves comfortable, since, of course, none of them wore clothes unless specifically instructed to do so by Mistress. Elise settled into the sofa with Todd, and they spoke to Sonja and hung out. An odd mix of normalcy and erotic display, chatting about the mundane moments of daily life and work while being served tea by nude slaves quietly passing through the heavy velvet curtain that separated kitchen and living room. Over the years, the cabin had come to feel like a home away from home for Elise. She and Sonja had known each other for so many years that it felt more like they were sisters than friends.

Sonja showed them to the guest bedroom, and Todd and Elise unpacked and waited for the night's play party to start. This would be the first time Todd would see Elise in her element, her sadism in full effect. It felt so intimate that he would see a side of her that few from her "normal" life ever would that it scared her. When she was in her dominance, truly connecting with the bottom, the room would fuzz into a soft focus until she could do nothing aside from working the body under her control, letting their howls roll over her skin and shudder through her bones. There could be a dozen people in the dungeon, but it was just her and the submissive in front of her. It excited her like nothing else when a sub's eyes opened wide with shock and fear as she moved unexpectedly from the lighter taps of a crop to the stinging, precise whacks that would land and leave rosy marks. Elise loved the idea that long after everyone left the cabin those marks would eventually bloom into bluish-green bruises—that her play partner for that evening would go about their life for the next few days with a reminder of her under their clothes.

Elise's attention jumped back to the present as she felt a familiar throbbing between her legs, the buzz of the here and now, the anticipation of the frenzied hedonism of this party. Later that night, as the party started, Todd respectfully watched and dabbled in activities that had, up until that point, just been fantasy for him. At brief moments, Elise could feel his gaze as he watched her in action, and she would flash a proud and lustful smile back at him. The buildup throughout the evening was excruciating until, when it was time to go to bed, Todd and Elise tore each other apart . . . landing in a tangled and sweaty pile of limbs.

The next morning Sonja would relay to all the partygoers that she'd had to reprimand the slaves to be quiet, as she'd wanted to listen to Todd's and Elise's orgasms. After everyone had had their breakfast and left the cabin, Todd and Elise stayed. It had been discussed in detail ahead of time and everyone's boundaries had been covered in case there was an opportunity to play. Todd had been understandably uncomfortable being objectified in public, even though it had been such a deep part of his private life. But now that the majority of the partygoers had gone, they had the opportunity to explore something new.

Sonja was in the basement surveying the slaves' cleanup from the previous night's festivities when Elise led Todd down the stairs to the dungeon. The same room, which had vibrated and heaved with energy just the night before, was now incredibly still. Elise locked eyes with Todd and told him plainly to undress. He jumped to comply, quickly disrobing as Sonja stared at them intently and climbed up to straddle a padded sawhorse. Elise ran her hands over his wide back, cupped his round ass, and asked if he was ready to serve. He eagerly nodded his head, looking wonderfully overwhelmed. Elise grabbed his cock and dragged him over to the sawhorse, forcefully bending him over and pushing him forward until his face was just out of reach of Sonja's crotch. Todd's breath shortened, his neck stretching forward to get just a little closer. Elise smacked his ass fast and hard and told him not to be a greedy little pig. She asked him to remember what his purpose was right now.

"Do you know your place?"

"Yes, Mistress, I'm yours to use in whatever way you wish."

"That's a very good answer, toy."

Elise started to slowly open Todd's ass with a plug, running her hands up and down his thighs while Sonja watched, and they giggled over him as he gasped and moaned. Elise put on her harness and strap and walked up to Todd, rubbed her lubed-up cockhead against the underside of his balls.

"Do you know what is about to happen, toy?"

"You're going to fuck me, Mistress?"

"Very presumptuous! Only if you are very good, toy."

His deep sigh and the relaxation of his body against the flat top of the sawhorse was subtle, but sweet. She poured more lube over his asshole and started to work the head of her cock inside him. He let out a gasp as she made that first stroke and his nose finally made contact with the silk-covered mound between Sonja's legs. She inched closer as Elise began to work Todd's ass, grabbing his hips and thrusting him forward until his face was completely buried between Sonja's thighs. Sonja and Elise smiled and nodded at each other over the back of this man's head and the wide expanse of his back—a man who was now just a delicious, faceless lump of flesh. It was what Elise had wanted all along. Sonja pulled aside her panties. You could hear Todd groan every time his face was pulled back from her wetness by Elise's grip and then pushed forward again into the damp pink of Sonja's pussy. Sonja grabbed Todd's ears and Elise kept her control over his hips as they used him like loggers use a saw. Time didn't seem to have any place in the dungeon. Elise got lost in her voyeurism as she watched Sonja writhing and tilting her head back while the toy's tongue flicked her clit. They eventually released him from this position once they'd had their fill. Elise stood him up and looked deeply into his eyes, taking in the blissful, serene look on his face. They sat down and she wrapped her arms around him and kissed his neck until he came back down to earth from subspace. Later that afternoon, as they pulled out of Sonja's driveway, Elise watched Todd navigate down the steep, curvy dirt road with her heart fluttering.

CHAPTER

# 17

# COSTUME BONDAGE

## Self-Discovery Through Costume Bondage

***By Mildred S. Pierce***

Costume bondage can assist in authentically creating a transformative experience for an individual who desires to don a particular submissive or dominant nature. Costuming can also tap into our deepest sexual human desires. In my personal experience, costume bondage and decorative masking have been used as a way to shield and protect my identity. Hiding my identity through decorative masking was also rooted in an attraction to hiding faces altogether. Even before my involvement with S/M dynamics, I created photographic images where eyes were bandaged up and hidden, faces were distorted or obsolete. I wish I had an understanding as to why I have an attraction to facelessness, but the heightened eroticism within my play dynamics is apparent when this aspect of decorative bondage comes into play.

Prior to understanding my sexuality and identity, it was a means of melding worlds together. Costume bondage, specifically face bondage and masks, opened my fascination with fetishism while still allowing me privacy. In the early stages of my involvement with the S/M community, I wore masks because I didn't yet accept my sexual desires due to preconceived shame. I was almost sex shaming myself. Decorative bondage created a sense of comfort to pursue scenes while having an aspect of anonymity. Since I am also passionate about photography, I enjoyed using photos as a means of documenting memorable scenes. Masking my face was important for hiding my identity, but also made it fun to look back on images and see what I refer to as the "faceless ghoul."

Over time, this sense of decorative face bondage and masking became an exciting aspect of play. How can my face be disguised this time? Is my partner interested in using vet wrap, rope braided into hair, or wrapping around the face? Can makeup and prosthetics be incorporated for creating an altered faceless identity? What aspect of decoration will enhance the scene and my personal enjoyment while succeeding in omitting the face?

Through all of this exploration, I discovered a new fetish: facelessness. Somehow, the realm of secrecy and staying hidden became a tool that not only created a scene persona, Mildred, but also introduced self-worth and empowerment to my play. Costume bondage evolved into a characteristic and personality trait of my scene identity, and also my personal life.

There is a fear of the unknown—it's daunting and ominous. Mildred's identity of being a "faceless ghoul," though, has generated a great sense of empowerment in my life. It has allowed me to evolve personally in my kink dynamics as well as in my daily life, because it relinquishes my dependence on identity. Developing an alter ego and character to represent an authentic and honest representation of myself has opened up more pure forms of identity. In current play scenarios or moments of intimacy, regardless of being a Top or a bottom, I try to actively continue having decorative bondage and masking incorporated into scenes. What started as a soothing or comforting practice evolved to create a realm of power dynamics and confidence. Even within my current photographic works, Mildred is always masked. Through facelessness, I can continue feeding into my own desires, even staying publicly hidden at events. Because Mildred is a faceless ghoul, she gets away with wandering around events while hiding in plain sight. I find this aspect to be incredibly entertaining.

Costume bondage is more than an exterior expression and form of artistic wrapping. Costume bondage can improve the psychological depths of an identity for expression through a kink persona. New fetishes may occur through deeper explorations and curiosities. Adding this element through my personal kink journey has improved play dynamics and fantasies that were never available when I was a beginner. The imagination can be heightened to new realms, incorporating new facets of understanding around your sexual desires. Adding decorative bondage into scenes can also create a new sense of self-acceptance and worth.

In my particular situation, omitting my face through decorative bondage allowed me to stop thinking about what I looked like and how other people were reacting, and become more focused on how I felt and my connection to my partners. Gimp masks made of vet wrap, latex hoods, lace masks, and face-altering accessories all gave me the ability to look through a different sensory-based context. Decorative face bondage allowed my play dynamics to heighten as well, because play became about incorporating other senses to experience the most important aspect of kink and scenes: the human connection and intimacy.

CHAPTER

# 18

# SENSATION BONDAGE

## Sensation Overload: A Rebirth

***By Mistress Couple***

The metal support beam in the center of the dungeon felt cold against my spine. I wondered how many people had been bound to it before. I had felt an electric charge when I first touched it, but wasn't sure if that was because of the beam itself or because of my nervous anticipation of what was to come. The play party had been in full swing for about two hours, and the scent of pheromones and sweat was thick in the air. The cracks of bullwhips, moans of sadomasochistic ecstasy, howls of pain, and exclamations of "Yes, Master," "Thank you, Mistress," "Please show mercy," and "PLEASE STOP OR I WILL COME" blended together into a symphony of erotic expression.

At the time, I was a slave in training, and had been instructed by my Master and Mistress to carry a small emerald under my tongue for the duration of the party. The exercise was meant to serve as a meditation on mental discipline and self-worth. With the emerald in my mouth, I was bound to the support beam while guests arrived for the party and curiously filtered into the dungeon. Mistress and one of her trainees, Blunt, had taken an industrial-size roll of plastic wrap and, starting at my feet, had wound it around me, securing me tightly to the pole.

"You're going to spend the entire party in this cocoon . . ." Mistress said in a soft, sultry voice. "I want you to get in touch with your inner beast. Use your senses. Let them feed you."

As she spoke, they continued to wind the plastic around my body, slowly engulfing me. The sticky film covered my knees and crept up my thighs. Blunt turned on a vibrator and instructed me to hold it between my legs, thrusting it into the gap between my thighs and jamming it into my clit. It wasn't like I had any other choice—I was stuck in that position—but I wasn't complaining about it one bit. As the wrap encircled my hips and touched the tip of the vibrator, the entire casing began to hum. Not only were my genitals beginning to pulse with lust, but my toes and ankles, the backs of my knees, every inch of my skin began to tingle and vibrate at the same frequency.

*Oh no . . .* I thought, *now I'm really in for it.*

"Now your body is set at the perfect frequency for erotic transformation," Blunt giggled, looking deeply into my eyes. The fact that she wasn't taking this whole procedure too seriously comforted me. I wasn't sure what erotic transformation was, or if I wanted it. All I knew was that I trusted my Mistress and Blunt's discretion and wanted to do what they asked.

As the plastic wound around my chest, it hugged me tightly to the support beam, making it difficult for my rib cage to expand. I worked on slowing down my breath so that I didn't panic. I could get enough air as long as I was patient about it. Master entered the dungeon with a sadistic glint in his eye, and my eyes darted fervently back and forth from his bulging leather codpiece to the two small cylinders he was holding in his hand.

"It's ziti . . ." he sardonically responded to my confused expression. "Ever had such a strange lifeline?"

"No, Master," I responded, still confused. What was he going to do with those noodles?

"Any last words?"

"Not besides thank you, Master."

"Okay, then . . . here you go, slavey . . ."

Before I knew it, the ziti noodles were each placed in one of my nostrils, and my face was tightly wrapped to the pole. The noodles poked out of the plastic to allow airflow. Not much, but just enough that I could maintain the predicament comfortably. The absurdity of the fact that I had noodles in my nose quickly disappeared, for they were the only things keeping me from suffocating. My breathing slowed even more.

There was a tap light placed by my right foot, and I was instructed to turn it on with my toe if I needed attention. The bondage was loose enough that it allowed for just enough movement to do so. Master, Mistress, Blunt, and the rest of the guests were now just a blur. Encased in the cocoon with the support beam vibrating against my spine, I was becoming less and less myself, and more and more part of the architecture. The party sprang into action around me, and I was left bound to the beam in the center of it all, instructed to absorb the energy of the evening using as many of my senses as I could.

With the permission of my Dominants (as well as my consent), party guests stopped to engage with me as they passed through the dungeon. The first thing I realized was that now that my vision was impaired, I had to try to identify who I was interacting with by the sound of their voice. The next thing I realized was how vulnerable I was. There I was, bound, vibrating, and naked but for the thin veil of plastic that covered me. Anyone could do whatever they wanted to do to me in that moment. Instead of panicking, I sucked on my emerald, thinking about how amazing it was that I had found a community that I trusted enough to share my body with in this way, and how much I wanted to share myself with them. I focused on the vibration that engulfed me. When someone touched me, I could feel the vibration transfer into their fingers, almost as if they were joining the union. Inside the cocoon, I buzzed away and continued to slip further into an erotic trance.

By this point, the erotic nature of the evening's activities and the restriction of my breath to the two small ziti tubes had joined forces in an olfactory assault. Mistress had sent a shy male slave over to tease my breasts, and as he warmed up from the initially hesitant light touch and progressed to pinching my nipples, I noticed that the pungent scent that had flooded my nostrils was morphing and shifting. Almost as if out of nowhere, I felt Master pressed up against the pole behind me, and heard him growling in my ear. The plastic wrap rattled against my right ear, vibrating as a result of Master's warm breath.

"Use your senses, slave. Arouse us. Learn what your slave brother's arousal smells like."

*Oh, so that's what's happening,* I thought. *They're teaching me how to use my senses to pick up on other people's states of arousal.*

The growling intensified, as did the nipple pinching. I continued to suck on the emerald. Continued to breathe. Continued to give of myself, and to take in my surroundings. Soon Master's cock was pressed up against my ass, and my slave brother's against my thigh. Both were humping and growling, breathing and scratching. As they continued, the scent transformed into a musky, thick, and incredibly intoxicating bouquet. On my next inhale, the scent was married with that of roses. Mistress must have also approached without me noticing.

"Hello, slave," she whispered into my left ear.

Yep. She was there, all right. The mashing together of bodies continued. Soon, we were all vibrating as one unit. The sounds and scents of the dungeon had melded with ours. I was starting to feel a warm tingling all over my body, starting at my toes and creeping toward my head, just as the plastic wrap had done.

"I'm going to count down from thirteen, and on one you may come, slaves," Master said.

"Thirteen . . . twelve . . . eleven . . ."

The tingling intensified.

"Ten . . . nine . . . eight . . ."

I began to shake.

"Seven . . . six . . . five . . ."

My teeth began to chatter.

"Four . . . three . . . two . . ."

*Oh Goddess, PLEASE hurry up!* I pleaded inside my head.

"ONE! COME, SLAVES!" he boomed.

Moans and wails filled the air. A rush of white light bounced through of every pore in my body and shot up toward the heavens from the crown of my head . . .

I'm not sure how long the chorus of orgasms lasted, or how long it took me to compose myself afterward, but as soon as I came to, I began to piece it all together.

*Oh . . . I see what they're doing her—*

Before I could finish my thought, I felt a sharp pain in my sternum. Mistress's talons were piercing the plastic. The tip of her nail felt like a knife as it tore through the plastic, splitting it open down the center of my body.

"Don't move," she ordered sternly.

A pair of safety shears were acquired by a slave, and the encasing around my face was carefully split up the center. The fuzzy outlines of people acquired more and more detail as my eyes adjusted to the light.

"Did you have a fun trip, slavey?" Mistress asked.

"Yes, Mistress. Thank you so much. Thank you all so much," I replied with a lump in my throat and tears forming in my eyes.

"Well, don't get all teary eyed yet. It's not over. You have one more thing to do," Master said in his usual sardonic tone.

"What's that?" I asked.

"Break free from your cocoon," said Blunt with a familiar grin as she flapped her arms. "Fly!"

Slowly, I lifted my arms, and the plastic that had been wrapped around me expanded like a pair of wings. If you'd asked me in that moment, I would have told you I was floating ten thousand miles above the dungeon.

While Blunt cleaned up the plastic, the male slave who had been pinching my nipples was instructed to wipe me down with cool, wet cloths. It had been hot in the cocoon, and I was covered in sweat. Eventually, I was brought upstairs, wrapped in a soft blanket, and instructed to put my emerald away somewhere safe and have something to eat. Cuddled up next to my leather family, I gluttonously shoveled fruit salad into my mouth, bringing my blood sugar back up to a normal level. The cinnamon flavor, which was usually so muted, overwhelmed my newly sensitized palate. I listened to the sounds of ecstasy continue to waft up from the dungeon and thought how my life would never be the same again. I truly had been transformed. My senses were more alive than they ever had been before, and therefore so was I.

CHAPTER

19

# FETISH BONDAGE

## Tension and Release

***By Mistress Couple***

**Trigger warning:** This essay contains anecdotes about my sexuality as a child. IN NO WAY do I endorse the sexualization of minors or pedophilia. The intent of sharing these intimacies with you, my reader, is to convey how a fetish is formed throughout childhood and adolescence.

My first balloon memory involves a failed bondage attempt. I couldn't have been older than three, and my parents had tied the balloon string around my wrist at the county fair. Faulty knot tying allowed it to break free and float away, heaven forfend! I actually don't remember anything about my emotional state about losing the balloon, although I assume I was pretty distraught. What I do remember was staring at the sky and watching the balloon get smaller and smaller as it floated away, the iridescent string fluttering in its wake. It truly was my first "one that got away"!

From the ages of four to nine, I became a pillow humper. I spent countless lazy Saturday mornings alone in my bedroom with my pillow "boyfriend," unbeknownst to any of my family members. I was mature enough to understand that what I was doing was "for adults" and that I should keep it a secret, but soon enough my parents walked in on me and put an end to my lazy Saturday mornings in bed. I was enrolled in all sorts of early-morning extracurricular activities—swimming, gymnastics, craft making—and while those activities got me out of bed, they did not rid me of my sexual fantasies. One Saturday evening, after a balloon-folding class taught by a local clown, I hid in my closet and twisted a folding balloon around my feet so that they couldn't move. I inflated a typical red balloon and drew a face on it. I named it Danny after John Travolta's character in *Grease*, who I had a huge crush on at the time. I was so excited about my imaginary bondage experience with a T-Bird that I didn't think through how I was going to escape, and thus after my imaginary balloon romp, the loud popping sound alerted my parents to the fact that I was still awake and up to no good. They rushed up to my bedroom and admonished me for being up past my bedtime. Looking back on the experience, I don't think they ever realized that what I was doing was sexual in nature, but being caught in the act of doing something sexual instilled me with a deep sense of shame and guilt. I vowed to stop playing sexual games with myself at home and to stop playing with balloons altogether. Something about them felt too lifelike.

In my teens, thanks to the invention of the internet, I started exploring my sexuality by watching pornography. I was surprised that most of the videos did nothing for me. In fact, most of them felt too contrived or violent and disturbing to me. I found three videos that I liked and felt that I would watch again and again. One was from the hard-core category and was a bondage sex video, but I didn't have the language to describe it as such at the time. The second was a gay male-on-male blow-job video. The third was a video of a man fucking a balloon and coming inside it. That was the one that I watched the most. I was fascinated by the image of the hard cock sliding in and out of the transparent rubber canal, and better yet, I was excited by it. I was relieved that I was not the only person in the world who had sexual feelings toward balloons. I also found those same feelings of childhood shame and guilt bubbling to the surface. I knew that what I had found was out of the ordinary in terms of sex, as I had found it listed under the "bizarre sex" category. I would obsess about the video, trying to prevent myself from going to the page and watching it, but eventually, hormones would win out, I'd go to the page, watch the video, and masturbate to orgasm. After the orgasm, I'd experience a deep emotional crash, overwhelmed by the guilt and shame that I was getting off on balloons. Was I sick? I didn't dare mention my balloon proclivity to anyone.

In my midtwenties, I began to explore BDSM and the fetish scene in New York City. I had arrived at the venue for my first New York City play party before my friends and was doing a loop around the club, taking in all the sights and sounds. There were many typical scenes that you'd expect at a fetish party—people being led around on leashes, spanked, flogged against St. Andrew's crosses—but in the middle of it all, one gentleman caught my eye. He was sitting on a bench, wearing a dalmatian mascot head with a firefighter's helmet, and blowing up balloons with a hand pump. My mind instantaneously flashed back to the images, tastes, and smells of my balloon boyfriend, and the lust I felt watching the balloon sex video. Did he know about that balloon porn video, too? Before I could stop myself, I was sitting next to the gentleman and asking him to explain his fetish to me. His eyes lit up at the prospect of an attractive young woman asking him to share, and he reached into his plastic bag, grabbing a transparent fourteen-inch balloon. He inflated the balloon quickly, tied it off with a knot, and placed it in my hands, but what he told me to do with it was completely different than what I expected.

"Close your eyes!" he said. "What do you feel?"

A giant grin appeared on my face. The balloon was pulsating

and vibrating. It was picking up the bass from the loud music blasting through the club's subwoofers and translating it into my hands.

"See, it's alive." He said as I opened my eyes to see him grinning back at me.

So I was right about Danny—it did feel real; the balloon took on a life of its own!

That was the beginning of a very special friendship with my first balloon fetish mentor. It turned out that Loonerdude had been one of the first-responder firefighters when the Twin Towers fell. Balloons were one of the only things in life that brought him joy and helped him through the depression that he experienced in the aftermath of that disaster. Being able to share that joy and teach others about it was incredibly special to him, and I was lucky enough to be a receptacle for all of the special knowledge that he had accumulated over the years. He started off by gifting me with my first balloon stash. Extralarge balloons that were dizzying to inflate, ribbed "worker" balloons, doughnut-shaped "geo-balloons" made especially for fucking, and even giant balloons that were large enough to climb inside!

He explained to me that we weren't sick. There was an entire community of balloon fetishists out there, and we were all stimulated by the metaphoric orgasmic tension and release that the balloons created. Some "looners" (balloon fetishists) eroticized the fear they experienced while inflating a balloon and anticipating the loud popping noise, others enjoyed the skin-like feel of the latex balloons. There were even folks who got off on the rubbery, musty taste of the balloons, and others still who became aroused by the sight of the bulging balloon with someone bouncing on it. Thanks to Loonerdude, I was able to explore my balloon fetish without the fear of being labeled as mentally unstable, but I was not able to shake the shame that I felt. After all, that shame had been ingrained in me since childhood. My dates with Loonerdude were swept under the rug and kept secret from most of my friends, and my balloon stash was exactly that. A stash, hidden away in the closet, just like Danny had been.

Last year, while at a BDSM conference, I attended a balloon fetish workshop. It was the first time that I was in a room with other balloon fetishists besides Loonerdude, and there must have been about twenty of us there. The enthusiasm in the room was palpable. It was clear that most of us had not spent time with other looners before, and the workshop quickly devolved into a giant balloon orgy! That was it. The dam burst. The shame I felt began to melt away and I started mixing balloon sex posts in with my other social media posts. By that point, with my reputation as a professional Dominatrix, my followers would not be surprised by my "eccentric" fetish.

Later in the year, while strolling through Prospect Park with a fellow Dominatrix friend, the subject of new sexual exploration came up. Her eyes widened, and with a curious grin she prodded, "So, I've been seeing on social media that you're getting into balloon sex. What's that all about?"

"Well," I said sheepishly, "I've actually been into balloon sex for years, I've just been too ashamed to share it with anyone. I've kept it really private, even from my partners."

"What? Why?"

"Well, you know, balloons are always associated with children, birthday parties, clowns . . . The general public just doesn't get it, so the balloon fetish community is constantly vilified and made fun of on internet forums. I guess I just didn't want to have to explain it or defend myself."

"I understand that, but Couple, basically the entire world knows that you have a human-size rotisserie spit in your backyard [and if they didn't, they do now!], and you're afraid of them knowing that you enjoy balloon sex? You *do* see how ridiculous that is, right?"

I did see it, and that ended the time period in which I was closeted about my balloon fetish. Now, I am broadcasting it for the world to read. I want other fetishists to know that they're not alone. I also want to clue others into why fetishism and "atypical" sex is so wonderful!

Over the past year or so, I've been delighted to introduce many friends and kinksters to the wonderful world of balloon sex. I've tied people up using folding balloons, encased them in my giant climb-in balloons, and even done breath play by forcing them to inflate a balloon to pop as quickly as they can. Each and every experience has been incredibly fun filled and playful. Each and every time, I worry that people are going to think that it's "too weird," but they come away with glazed eyes, aroused genitals, and exclamations of "YES. I GET IT NOW," or "Uh-oh! I think you just turned me into a looner!" Owning and sharing your fetishes can be an incredibly liberating and empowering experience; at least it has been for me. I guess what I'm trying to say is that a fetish can become bondage if you don't express it. Forget the tension—it's all about the release.

CHAPTER

# 20

# SENSORY-DEPRIVATION BONDAGE

## The Ultimate Supplication

***By patient of Mistress Tess NYC***

One aspect of bondage that is often overlooked is hydrotherapy. Prior to the advent of psychotropic drugs, violent mental patients were often restrained for hours in specially constructed circulating bathtubs with canvas top sheets restricting their movement. After the warm bath, patients were frequently placed in ice-cold wet sheets to further calm them. Many Tops have subjected their bottoms to such therapy in recent years.

After reading the accounts of such treatments, I asked my Mistress to try it. She thought it quite kinky and accommodated my request.

It started out in a Jacuzzi, where I was placed in a canvas body bag. The circulating warm water relaxed me, and I was unable to move a muscle. My private parts were exposed, and my Mistress teased and denied me both manually and with waterproof vibrators. My anal region was likewise titillated. This went on for hours. At the moment I thought I would explode, she would stop, let me regroup, and start all over again. It was incredible to be helpless and at her mercy. To add to the realism she wore a very sexy white nurse's uniform.

After what seemed like an eternity, I was transferred to a table with five ice-cold sheets. I was forced to lie down, faceup, on the first sheet, where I started to freeze. The contrast between the warm Jacuzzi and first wet sheet was incredible. The top sheet was snugly fit to my body. A second, third, fourth, and fifth sheet were added. I was mummified. Initially I froze. The sheets hugged my body like a glove. A blanket was placed over all the sheets, followed by saran wrap and then a restraint sheet. Belts further secured this arrangement. An inflated rubber body bag encased this elaborate restraint system. I couldn't move a single body part. It was so intense. A rubber inflatable hood was added, and ropes through its D rings further secured my head. I was then suspended off the table. The weight of the sheets was overpowering, and absolutely no movement was possible. This included my shoulders, arms, toes, and eyebrows. I lay there blowing in the wind. Holes were precut for the genitals, and electrodes were placed so the electrical stimulator box could do its work. The waves, ramps, and all programs of the "box" were relentless. I had a vibrating anal plug inserted. A hands-free masturbation device was set on a slow speed, and I was edged for hours. At the moment I thought I would release, my mistress stopped the teasing and denial, refusing me any release. Interestingly, my body temperature rose reflexively and I no longer felt cold, despite still being wrapped in wet sheets. The feeling of total supplication and surrender was complete. Mistress and I had agreed on a policy of consensual nonconsent, so there was no way for me to escape, and truthfully, I didn't want to.

When you are placed in wet sheets, your mind is focused only on submission and survival. You realize more than ever before that there is simply no way out. You are at your Mistress's mercy. Body bags, straitjackets, collars, and hoods are restrictive but not paralyzing. The wet sheets provide the sense of total supplication. There is simply no movement except the chest wall and the genitals (when they are sensually stimulated). Adding the electrics is not dangerous, since the area is relatively dry and the current is bipolar. Still, the patient has to have total confidence in his nurse's competence and training and must trust that nothing "bad" will happen—in my case, Mistress had trained herself extensively on the possible risks of the scenario and signs that my body might be in trouble, and I knew I could trust my safety to her.

In this kind of scene, you are there for your Top's pleasure and your therapy. When you are brought to different arousal states, it is the ultimate mind/body experience because you cannot move your fingers, arms, legs, and toes. Your abdomen is secured. Chest excursion is at the mercy of your therapist, and how much air you will be allowed is in her hands. As you lie there, the sensation of genital pleasure is coupled with the reality that nothing you do will change the outcome. You are usually gagged, so verbal requests are out of the question. However, if your nurse keeps reinforcing your predicament and dropping hints on what is yet to come . . . how could anything be more restricting or mind blowing?

* BDSM practitioners should never attempt a consensual nonconsent scene, especially one involving breath restriction, without training by experienced practitioners and professionals.

CHAPTER

# 21

# PREDICAMENT BONDAGE

## An Erotic and Fearsome Tale

***By Karin Webb (aka Creature)***

The predicament itself came from holding my body in a stressful position at the end of a long night's scene with a very large hunting knife roped between my legs, threatening my pussy at the slightest give in to relaxation.

I had met my play partner earlier that day. We were both teaching workshops at a fetish convention, and he stumbled into one of my classes, which I was demo bottoming for: Food Play 101. It turns out licorice rope makes a mean whip, but that's not the point of this story . . .

I was relatively new to sadistic Dominants back then, though no stranger to my own masochistic tendencies. The buzzing high I got from a sound beating, the release of sexy warmth from blood play, the ecstatic knowledge that my body was solely and completely my own to challenge as I wished, and the desire to give myself over to someone bigger than I in order to survive were all testaments to my love of pain. We met that night in the dungeon. I stripped sensually and with confidence under his amused and complimentary gaze. This strange man ran me through an assortment of new-to-me tricks. I discovered being whipped wasn't as scary or painful as I thought it would be, something I would spend multiple hours enjoying one future day—but that isn't the point of this story, either . . .

His fingers were knowledgeable in pressure points, and I became his naked rag doll–puppet, dancing, crumpling, and moving at his whim. There was a fair amount of punching, and his heavily booted feet introduced my body to the bass resonance of being kicked. The contents of his toy bag emptied, and along with the fresh sting of his whip, floggers dragged heavily on my backside, paddles marked my thighs, canes of various thicknesses and flexibilities striped me, even a martial arts iron fan opened loudly (making me jump), and when struck closed, lashed out quickly, its solid violence imprinting painfully.

This man had, from our beginning, the desire to find an edge of mine and own it. His sadism was not just physical but also mentally attuned, and he hadn't satisfied the latter curiosity yet. At some point I absentmindedly pulled my leg over my head to stretch. Partners have not infrequently commented on my dancer's flexibility and strength. He grabbed the opportunity.

Seconds after my leg came down, I found myself flipped onto my back on a table and growled at to lift my hips. Head and shoulders on the table, feet underneath me, and my midsection lifted toward the ceiling, I formed a bridge pose and was tied firmly there. Below my bare ass, a large hunting knife appeared, the kind you gut animals with or show off in order to intimidate a larger foe. My heart skipped a beat seeing its shiny tip below me, and it was secured at such a height and angle that if I let my hips fall, even just a little . . . well . . . the knifepoint, closely and squarely aimed toward my vulva, would push farther into me, threatening to slice me open wider where I already split.

Having never been in such a predicament before, I was nonplussed at first. I was disturbed and wary of the situation I found my most private body in, but confident in my strength. In that particular pose, my thick ballet-trained thighs can keep up for days. He mused out loud about how long he thought I could hold my position before having my pussy bloodied. The low estimate he uttered enticed a cocky grin to my lips, and I brightened, thinking how easy it would be to win this round of our games. What I did not know was that this Dominant, who had been switching up activities all evening, flitting between this new idea and that new toy, could also wait.

And wait . . .

And wait . . .

And wait.

Two minutes became four, and then seven, ten . . . twenty? I lost track somewhere after that. Time became meaningless in the rising tide of my masochistic euphoria. Determined not to fold, my will switched into high gear, proving my physical strength, which I'd developed in the discipline of letting my body's needs go as I maintained a peaceful sense inside. I persisted. Every time my hips dipped a little in momentary relaxation, I felt cold metal and the knife's tip swing in tighter to touch the sides of its new sheath, my vagina, warning me not to relax any further. Time ticked by and my partner made no move to release me . . .

The dungeon at this convention was enormous, and my sadistic friend waved over this acquaintance and that to take a look: knife centered on my vulva, hips defying gravity, time marching on while kinkster after kinkster shook their heads or arched their eyebrows and laughed out loud. He repeated over and over again, almost deliriously, what a crazy sub I was to let him—a strange man—do this to me. He was giddy at the violence of our situation. Asking me, "Aren't you getting tired after so long straining?" Reminding me, "Be careful not to let yourself fall on that knife because of overexertion." Whispering hotly in my ear, "There's no shame in calling red." He mused loudly and often about how bloody my pussy would be if I shifted, and cooed at how much pain must be mounting in the stiff muscles of my struggling body.

What felt like hours after I should have worn out, my legs started trembling and he laughed, poking more fun at my expense, repeating what a crazy sub I was to let him play with my body this way. I started to worry, those familiar perseverations of "What have I gotten myself into?" and "What will my mother think when she sees the body?" started overtaking my mental sanctity. Slight trembling became visible shaking, and he asked me what color I was at. I changed my tune from the casual "green" I had been yawning at him to a dry, thin, labored "yellow," and he told me how sexy I was. He said how turned on this scene had made him, and that it was too bad we had negotiated no sex because he was very, very hard for me right now. He wasn't ready to let me go just yet.

More time, shaking, and now sweating, too. Torn between pleasing him and being honest about my own strength and boundaries, I was turning the word *red* over and over in my mind, trying to figure out in which moment it would jump from my mouth to end it all. More and more frequently the knife's end became acquainted with my inner lips, scraping back and forth. I was playing "just the tip" with a strange man's weapon. He was fucking me with anxiety and penetrating my pain-ridden body without the slightest touch.

To this day, I don't remember if I said "red" out loud or not. I was deep in the heavy fog of trembling, sweating, pain-processing subspace. Just as I felt myself give in to the idea of ending everything, though, warm hands steadied me between the thighs. He pulled back the handle of his knife and flashed it from below. I stayed in position, unmoving. Hips in the air, legs sweating and shaking, I locked eyes with him. An impressed smile spread across his lips, and sparkling, impish love radiated toward me. "You did really well, Creature. Come down now. You may relax."

Permission granted.

The spell of this physical challenge and our emotional wrestling: undone.

My ass and thighs released their tense hold of my torso, and I melted like molasses to the tabletop, exhausted and shivering. I was proud, seeing the pleased affections on my sadistic friend's face. We kissed passionately and then tenderly; he blanketed me and curled up beside me. Warm and wrapped in his embrace, quiet, I felt a deeper release shudder out from inside. Slow tears slid from my eyes. "How fucked-up am I?" I thought. My body had taken so much, yet I felt more real, more alive, more turned on and satisfied than ever; I felt more equal to and more seen by this strange man who had pounded on me, challenged, calculatedly endangered, relentlessly taunted, and exhausted me than pretty much anyone I had ever fucked at that point in my life. My tears admitted the fear that I am broken, and I was caught for a moment judging myself. What did it mean that I would go to such extremes to stay present and feel wanting sensually? What was this illness?

As I entertained these thoughts, they evaporated like my silent tears back into nothing. No, I realized, there isn't anything broken. I feel alive and present because I survive. I'm grateful to have this body, to be played with and challenged by partners imaginatively and consensually, who listen to the wanting creature deep inside me. My fear and shame dissipated, and for the first time I beautifully understood: I am kinky.

CHAPTER

22

# SUSPENSION BONDAGE

## Finding and Holding My Space

***By Do***

I have always loved bondage. Ever since I first delved into the world of BDSM—over ten years ago—the feel of restraints has always been intensely erotic to me. Collars. Cuffs. Chains. Leather straps. Silk scarves. And, of course, rope.

Rope is special. So many weights, textures, shapes, sizes. It can torment, tease, arouse, and subdue. And, it can elevate. Literally.

I've only been suspended a few times. Like so many people, I wondered what it would be like to fly. The first time I was suspended, I remember the moment my feet left the ground . . . and I thought, *Oh . . . this is what it's like.*

Suspension for me is a delicacy and a privilege—something that I enjoy rarely. It's not something I want to do with just anyone. Recently I found that I wanted—I needed—to be suspended. I needed to fly. To be wrapped up in rope . . . and pulled and twisted and turned . . . and to soar. To float.

Fortunately, the perfect person and place were headed my way.

One of the guest masters for a La Domaine Esemar party was a rigger I knew and trusted. He'd tied me before. I wasn't able to approach him until the afternoon before the party. I almost didn't have to finish the request before he agreed. His answer was something to the effect of, "Oh, absolutely. It'll happen. Count on it." I was excited. And I was, oddly enough, scared. He ties in a challenging fashion. I knew that the tie would be tough. I have a tendency to panic when there is no reason to. *Don't do that tonight*, I told myself. *This is working out because it's supposed to work out. You want this and you need this. See it through. Don't work against yourself.*

He taught a bondage workshop that afternoon. I sat in on some of it. He did some beautiful, complex ties. I saw slaves with their limbs stretched and strained and twisted. The rope wrapped around them like beautiful clothing, making them look their best. They looked sexy. Special. Graceful. Would I look like that? Could I look like that?

*Don't be disappointed if it doesn't happen*, I told myself. *You've been tied by him before. There are people here who want to be tied by him for the first time. Don't be selfish. Be a grown-up.*

As the party swung into action, I sat on the dungeon floor talking to one of the masters in training. I watched scenes start, connections made, and felt the sexual, kinky buzz build. Across the dungeon I watched the rigger set up for the evening. As I watched him unpack his rope and hang the ring, I got more and more excited. And nervous.

He walked across the dungeon to where I was sitting. He looked at the suspension setup, then at me, then back at the setup, then back at me.

*Oh*, I realized. *Now. It's going to happen now.*

I excused myself and followed him. Since the last time he tied me, I'd developed some issues with my right knee. I made sure he knew what my knee could and couldn't take. He nodded in understanding.

Then he asked me, "So what do you want? Easy? Or rough?"

Hmm . . . I wasn't expecting that. I chose option C.

"Could you do somewhere in between?"

"Sure, no problem."

I got into position—which for me means standing up straight, weight equally balanced, and my hands on the back of my head. (The times I've been tied that I haven't used good posture . . . not good. In fact, very bad and very uncomfortable.) He picked up the rope and began.

He seemed to tie me very quickly. The rope went around my chest. My waist. My legs. Between my legs. I felt covered and cocooned. And the nerves grew. *Breathe*, I kept telling myself. *Just breathe.*

He kept in close contact with me. He pulled me back against him to place the ropes. He lifted body parts as he needed to. He seemed to do this at just the right times. When I felt him close, I remembered, *You know him. You care for him and he cares for you. You're safe. He's got you.*

As he tied me, he said, "Not tonight, but another time, I'll tie you rough. That time, you'll have to crawl out of here." Hearing that aroused me. That kind of tie . . . that kind of experience . . . the pain . . . the sensuality . . . yes, I wanted and needed that. But not tonight.

I don't remember the position I was in when I left the ground. I don't remember how many positions he put me in. But there is one position that I remember very well.

I was turned over onto my stomach. I was facing down toward the dungeon floor. I had a perfect view of the party and of nearly everyone in that particular part of the dungeon. I saw two of the people I love most in the world—Master R and Mistress Couple—below me. I heard and saw and felt others in the La Domaine family. I heard and saw and felt the other guests—people who were at different points in their journey through BDSM.

As I was cradled in the ropes, I felt myself spread out and open up. My body adjusted to the tension and pull of the ropes.

I felt my mind, my consciousness, open up as well. I could feel my family. My friends. My coworkers. And on and on. I could feel all the elements of my life . . . yet I was above them and outside them. I could feel the ropes biting at me . . . yet I could hardly feel them at all. It was an extraordinary moment. I felt the connections . . . yet I was outside them.

It was overwhelming at times. *Breathe*, I remembered. *Let it happen.* I let the emotions and the connections flow over and around and through me. I can be part of this, I realized. I can be part of all this and still be me. I don't need to give everyone my everything. I can give, but I can still be me. I can still hold space for myself.

All too soon, it was time to come down. My feet hit solid ground. The ropes came off. And the party went on.

I floated through the rest of the night. I was very present, very active. But the suspension stayed with me. I felt calm. Serene. Yet I felt energized. Empowered. Whole.

This experience clarified for me that I need structure to be free. I need to be pushed and challenged in order to grow. I need to honor my connections without letting them drag me down. I can step outside the network of my life and look at all of it, be part of it, be present, and yet still have a private and personal self. I am a slave, a Domme, a sister, a daughter . . . but I am not just those things. I'm all of those things and many more.

That night was a key point in my relationship with bondage. I don't believe it is the high point. A high point, but not the high point. Life takes twists and turns and wraps and bites . . . just like rope. We'll see where I end up next.

CHAPTER

# 23

# SELF-BONDAGE FOR ONE AND TWO

## Self-Bondage

### *By Master R*

### *Self-Bondage for One: The Beginning*

I started tying myself because I had no one else to tie. Think about that. With that motivation, at the initial moment of creation, it was, first and foremost, the act of a Dominant. As I selected the rope, I thought about the cock and balls I was about to torment in brand-new clothesline. I considered what those bulging balls, what that tightly wrapped erect cock would feel like in my hands. I considered how I would squeeze and twist my own sex until my victim desired nothing but mercy and orgasm. My testosterone flowed and mixed with my dominance—governed by the line I held and was about to brutally apply.

It all changed when I put the rope around the base of my cock and balls and sadistically went to make a very cutting and very tight square knot. I drew hard on the working end of the line, with my dominance thinking about what that must feel like to the one being tied—and then I felt it. As the rope tightened, my paradigm shifted and I was suddenly the submissive in the arrangement. I felt the blood engorging my penis, blood trapped by the tightness of the bondage at the base of my sex, and at that moment, felt the bondage throughout my sexual being. Fully aroused, I realized that masochism was now coursing through me. I wanted, I needed, someone to slap my tied cock. I wanted that stimulation to arouse me and force me tighter and tighter into the bonds. And I wanted to feel as if the fate of my tightly tied cock and balls lay in someone else's hands.

I looked down at the predicament I had created. I saw a slave's organs, waiting to be hurt. Instantly, the dominance I felt when I first reached for the rope surged back into me. I had a beautiful cock in front of me, all tied up and begging to be hit. I grabbed the patterned rope in my left hand and gave a strong, dominant pull, forcing the slave to let out a small gasp of surprise and pain. Suddenly, my self-bondage took me once again into the realm of submission, and I felt the hand of a Master slap my sex, over and over. I grew even larger in the ropes—ropes I had inflicted upon myself. I encouraged my Master to hit me harder. The ropes that I held in my dominant hand grew ever tighter on my still engorging cock. I looked again at my balls, and they were slave's balls. I hit them as a Master with a tied slave, and I felt the blow as the tied slave I had just become.

I felt the dizzying power of orgasm approaching. I felt the sensual excitement of having a tied slave nearing orgasm. I teased the slave again and again, knowing the rope would hold me, that there was no escaping this self-motivated beating.

Put another way, self-bondage allows me to be Master and slave simultaneously. Life is sweet, *n'est-ce pas*?

### *Self-Bondage for Two*

Home alone. Very horny. Ring cell phone, ring. At last. Mistress's most dulcet voice. "Slave, I will be home at five thirty. I want you on the bed, fully restrained, at 5:25, cock and balls tied imaginatively and stretched to the ceiling, ropes tied to ankle cuffs, ropes tied to wrist cuffs. Nipples weighted and pulling to your sides. You may choose three toys that you will have lying by your side when I arrive."

I start with the cuffs. I open the bottom drawer to my dresser and intake the smell of the leather. I select the cuffs. I find the locks. As I wrap the first ankle cuff around my leg and lock it in place, I start to arouse myself. One more ankle cuff. Breath becomes heavier. The first wrist cuff takes me closer into a vortex, swirled by my close desires and her still distant ones. The first wrist cuff locks, and the locking binds me to her. The second embraces my wrist, and the lock secures our lust. Cuffed. Even with the cuffs not yet secured to a post or a pillar, they have immediately added the extraordinary and powerful element of Mistress restraining my psyche.

Now comes tying the cock and balls—with imagination. I know I can use my imagination; I wonder how I can use hers.

Start with the basics. A rope around the base of my sex, tied with tight love and a square knot. Then I wrap each ball separately and out to the side. Right one first, with four, now five wraps of rope; left one next, four or five wraps of rope, and now my balls are separated far apart from each other. I continue with the rope, up and down my cock, knotting at each level up and each level back down. At the base again, I take what is left of the line and I wrap it around my balls from above, pulling them over the top of my hard cock. I tie them in place like that; they can go nowhere. They are totally vulnerable in this state. It is now time to go find the three toys Mistress has requested. I lay them on the bed, to the far side of where I will soon be restraining my rampant sexuality.

The nipple clamps are easy. Stretching the cock and balls to the ceiling for Mistress, not so easy. I opt for a five-pound weight on a rope that will run through an eyelet in the ceiling, and then down to my body, where I will weave the rope into the tie around my now darkening cock and balls. Before I do that deed, I must secure my ankles. There are four ropes, one on each corner of the bed. I stretch my legs and run a line through the eyelet on the right leg's cuff. I tie it off with a quick-release knot, and then I repeat the process with my left leg. As soon as I lie back and secure my wrists, the knots will become inescapable, but Mistress will be able to remove them with ease. Now, with legs spread and tied, I set the weight. When the weight is hanging, I feel a deeply submissive float taking over my body. I continue by locking my left wrist to its appropriate rope line. I stretch and twist my now 95 percent restrained body until, with the help of a short piece of chain and a Master lock, I manage to get my right arm securely restrained. I am in a trap of my own making. I am a widely spread eagle. I am wildly excited and fully anticipatory. There is no escape.

I feel my legs pulled apart. I feel my stretched cock and balls, throbbing in the direction of the ceiling. I can no longer reach the clamps that are now beginning to make my nipples sore and eroticized. I have no choice but to submit to this pain that Mistress so lovingly requested, and that I inflicted. I look at the clock. It is 5:24. There is nothing I can do now but give in to the bondage, the arousal, the growing passion, and wait to hear Mistress's dulcet voice at five thirty.

Well, this is your last stop! We've come to the end of our journey together. I hope that throughout the course of reading this book you have learned a great deal both about bondage and about yourself. I know that throughout the course of writing it, I have.

Keep in mind, as with many other things in life, the most important part of exploring bondage is the journey, not the destination. Be patient with yourself and your partners. Stay curious, stay careful, stay focused, and stay hungry. Goddessspeed and good luck in your exploration.

# NOTES

***Notes for Chapter 1:***

"Dictionary of Sex Terms," *Kinkly* (blog), accessed September 9, 2017, https://www.kinkly.com/dictionary.

Wikipedia, s.v. "BDSM", last modified May 26, 2018, 16:59, https://en.wikipedia.org/wiki/BDSM.

GLBTQ Encyclopedia (archive), "Leather Culture," by Matthew D. Johnson, accessed November 17, 2017, http://www.glbtqarchive.com/ssh/leather_culture_S.pdf.

Sam Dylan Finch, "Ever Been Told to 'Check Your Privilege?' Here's What That Really Means," *Everyday Feminism* (blog), July 27, 2015, https://everydayfeminism.com/2015/07/what-checking-privilege-means/.

Kashiko Black, "Kink & BDSM Ethics: Morality When Inflicting or Receiving Pain," *Keeping It Kinky* (blog), April 6, 2015, http://www.keepingitkinky.net/bdsm/kink-basics/ethics/.

***Notes for Chapter 2:***

Kirigami. "Shibari VS Kinbaku," *Rope Tales* (blog), accessed November 20, 2017, https://www.ropetales.com/shibari-vs-kinbaku/.

"Rope Selection," Knot Right Supply LLC, accessed September 20, 2017, http://www.knotrightsupply.com/info/rope-selection/.

### *Notes for Chapter 3:*

Wikipedia, s.v. "Key (Lock)," last modified May 13, 2018, 03:12, https://en.wikipedia.org/wiki/Key_(lock).

"The Heretic's Fork," *Torture Museum* (blog), accessed October 17, 2017, http://torturemuseum.net/en/the-heretics-fork/.

Brad Smithfield, "Scold's bridle—The gruesome medieval torture instrument worn to deter women from gossiping," *The Vintage News* (blog), May 5, 2016, https://www.thevintagenews.com/2016/05/05/scolds-bridle-the-gruesome-medieval-torture-instrument-worn-to-deter-women-from-gossiping/.

### *Notes for Chapter 4:*

Daniel, "Erotic Hypnosis—What It Is, and Why You Should You [*sic*] Try It," *Hypnotic Dreams* (blog), November 10, 2017, https://www.hypnoticdreams.com/erotic-hypnosis/.

### *Notes for Chapter 5:*

Mark Griffiths, "Horsing around: A beginner's guide to pony-play." Dr. Mark Griffiths (blog), July 6, 2012, https://drmarkgriffiths.wordpress.com/tag/the-aristotelian-perversion/.

"House of Gord: The Home of Ultra Bondage," accessed December 8, 2017, https://www.houseofgord.com/.

### *Notes for Chapter 6:*

"The History of the Wedding Band," With These Rings, accessed October 2, 2017, http://withtheseringshandmade.com/history-of-wedding-rings/.

"Waist Training vs Tight Lacing—What's the Difference?" *Lucy's Corsetry* (blog), October 13, 2013, https://lucycorsetry.com/2013/10/13/waist-training-vs-tight-lacing/.

John Willie, *The Adventures of Sweet Gwendoline* (New York: Bélier Press, 1999).

### Notes for Chapter 7:

"Sexual Masochism Disorder," *Psychology Today*, March 6, 2018, https://www.psychologytoday.com/conditions/sexual-masochism-disorder.

### Notes for Chapter 9:

"5 Types of Brain Waves [*sic*] Frequencies: Gamma, Beta, Alpha, Theta, Delta," *Mental Health Daily* (blog), April 15, 2014, https://mentalhealthdaily.com/2014/04/15/5-types-of-brain-waves-frequencies-gamma-beta-alpha-theta-delta/.

Biotele, "Ganzfeld: Hack Your Brain the Legal Way," *Instructables* (blog), March 7, 2009, http://www.instructables.com/id/Ganzfeld-Hack-Your-Brain-the-Legal-Way/.

### Notes for Chapter 10:

Shin Nawakiri, *Essence of Shibari Kinbaku and Japanese Rope Bondage* (Lynwood: Mystic Productions LLC, 2017).

### Notes for Chapter 11:

"Like Ra's Naughty Playground," accessed December 15, 2017, https://www.likera.com/home.php.

David Stein, "Doing It Yourself," *AltSex* (blog), 1995, https://web.archive.org/web/20021202101120/http://www.altsex.org/bdsm/self-bd-1.html.

# ACKNOWLEDGMENTS

This book is dedicated to those who cleared the path before me and guided me to the place where I could write this book, as well as those who will follow after me and forge their own paths. May your legacies and journeys be rich and rewarding!

Writing this book has been a truly magical experience. The project has transformed from "my book" into a book that my community helped bring to fruition. I felt so loved and supported throughout this process, and I am eternally grateful for the alchemy that occurred here.

To my partner and mentor Master R, who kept my body and soul nourished during this challenging process.

To the La Domaine leather family, who offered your bodies and minds as the testing grounds for this book, specifically Do, Blunt, Rocky, Quest, 9, destiny, slice, hum, Gage, Flower slave, and Librarian slave.

To New Orleans, specifically, Beatrice, Eli, Smudge, Creature, Dayna, Winter Palace, and all of its inhabitants for your love, support, and magical manifestation.

To all those who beautified the book with their artwork: Kiki, Emily. And all involved in the photo shoot: Oz, Cassavini, Duchess Jealoquin, Lady M, Mildred, Gage, Rocky, Quest, 9, hum, slice, Amanda, and Simone.

To all those who fortified the book with their writing: Andi, Do, Claire Hex, destiny, Mildred, Domina Franco, Creature, slave of Tess, Master R, and Daemonumx.

To my bondage mentors: Master R, Mistress Collette, Master Max, Murphy Blue, Marcuslikesit, David Lawrence, Gorgone, Lee Harrington, and KissMeDeadlyDoll.

To Hannah, Meghan, Sara, Allyson, and the rest of the Cleis Press staff for giving me this opportunity and believing in my vision.

To all those I haven't mentioned who asked "How's your book coming along?" I appreciated that more than you know!

Thank you to my blood family for putting in the work to understand me and my path and for supporting it, especially when it is difficult.

Last but never least, this book is dedicated to those who remain in non-consensual bondage. Until all of us are free, none of us truly are.

Printed in the United States
By Bookmasters

Printed in the United States
By Bookmasters